an introduction to
HOMEOPATHY

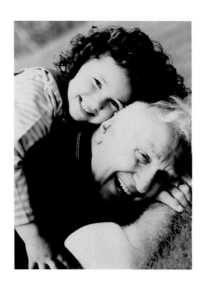

p

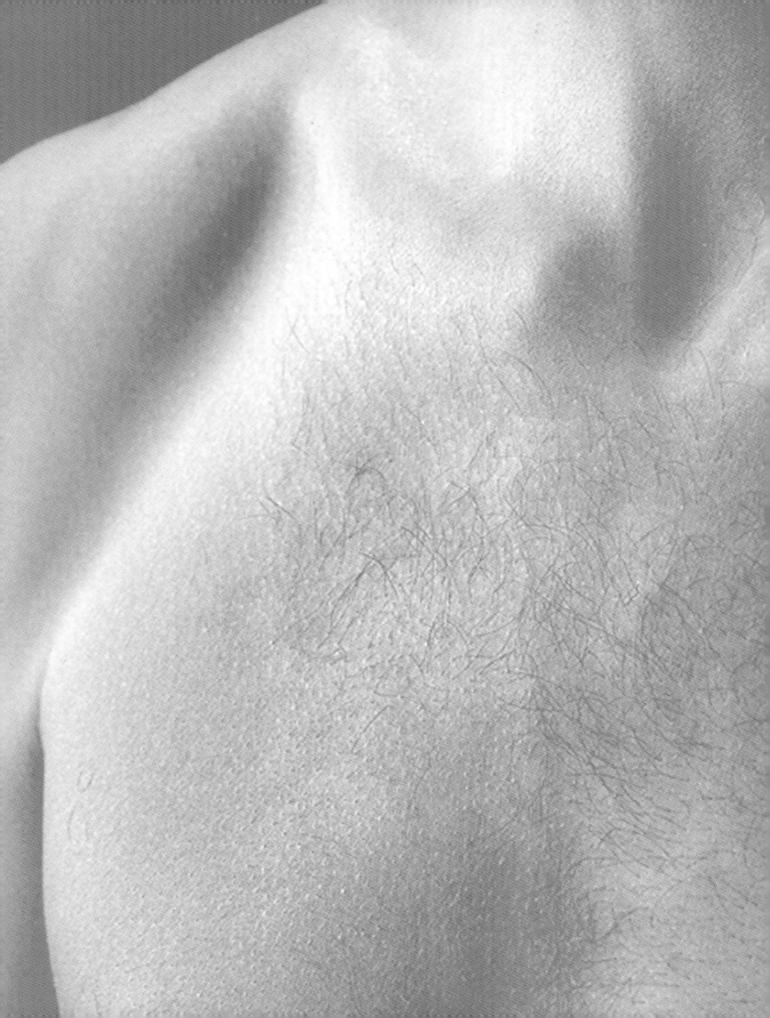

an introduction to
HOMEOPATHY

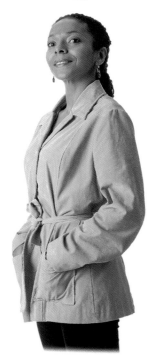

Rima Handley

This is a Parragon Publishing book
First published in 2002

Parragon Publishing
Queen Street House
4 Queen Street
Bath BA1 1HE, UK

This book was created by
THE BRIDGEWATER BOOK COMPANY

Art Director: Stephen Knowlden
Designers: Chris and Jane Lanaway
Editorial Director: Fiona Biggs
Project Editor: Lizzy Gray
Picture Research: Trudi Valter and Vanessa Fletcher

ISBN 1-84273-438-5

Manufactured in China

Contents

Homeopathy defined   6

What is **homeopathy?**   8

The **origins** of **homeopathy**   10

The **development** of **homeopathy**   12

What is a **remedy?**   14

Principles and **practice**   16

Understanding
symptoms and **remedies**   18

The **complete** picture   20

Types of **illness**   22

Homeopathy in **action**   24

Identifying symptoms   26

Finding the **remedy**   32

Giving or **taking** remedies   34

Waiting for the **remedy** to work   36

Materia Medica   38

Directory of common **ailments**   72

Case **histories**   88

Useful addresses   94

Index   95

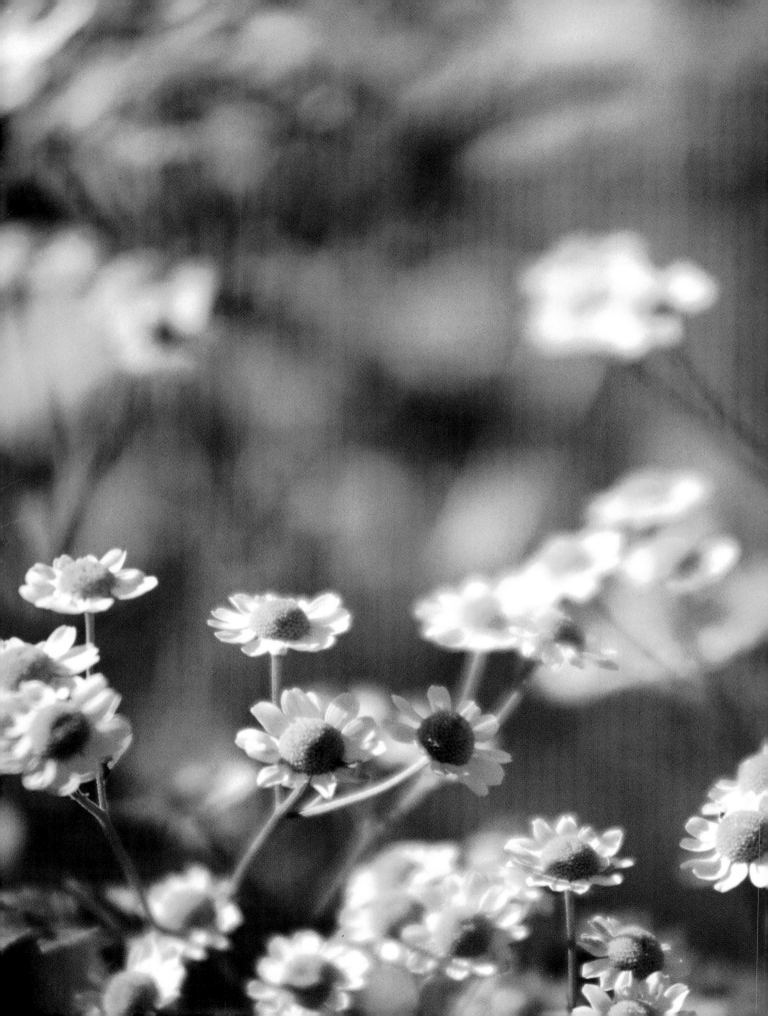

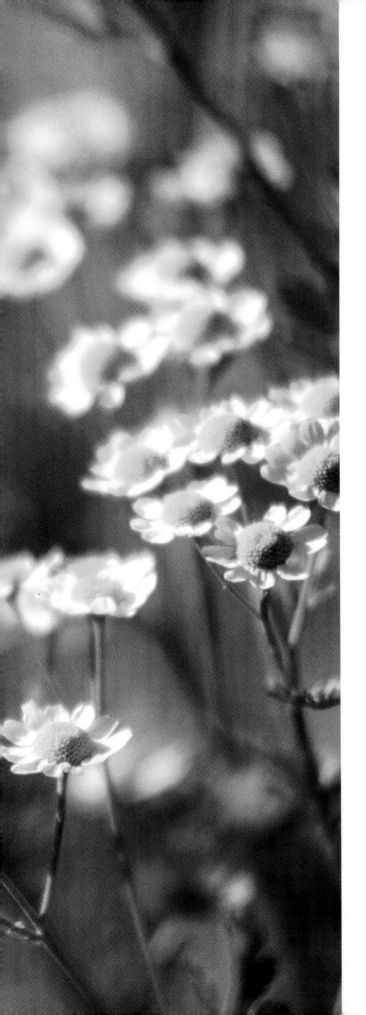

Homeopathy defined

Developed by Samuel Hahnemann over 200 years ago, homeopathy is a gentle, yet effective form of natural healing. By harnessing the power of different organic substances—flowers, animals, minerals—remedies are developed to work in harmony with the body to fight many common ailments and diseases.

What is **homeopathy?**

Homeopathic medicine has been in existence for more than 200 years. It was 1786 when Samuel Hahnemann, the German doctor who discovered and developed it, put into words homeopathy's basic first principle: *similis similibus curentur*, or "like cures like." In so doing, he turned on its head the ideas behind orthodox medicine. Orthodox medicine, or "allopathy," doesn't use "like to cure like"—it treats illness with something different.

German physician Samuel Hahnemann (1755–1843) was the founder of homeopathy.

Homeopathy cures by treating a sick person with substances (remedies) that actually bring about a very slight exaggeration of the symptoms of the original illness. In this way, it encourages the body's healing system to throw off both the original disease and the artificially added disease. This is why the term "homeopathy" was used: it comes from the Greek *homoi* (similar) and *pathos* (suffering). This is in direct contrast to allopathy (orthodox medicine): the word "allopathy" come from the Greek *allo* (other or different) and *pathos* (suffering).

Homeopaths believe that the human body is always trying to keep itself healthy and in balance. When health is under threat from harmful external forces such as bacteria, viruses, and stress, or from internal forces such as genetic predispositions, the body produces symptoms such as pain, cough, or fever in an attempt to restore a healthy balance. Fever, for example, is part of the body's attempt to deactivate a virus, and mucus is an attempt to expel invading material from the body. Homeopathy seeks to support these symptoms and encourage them rather than suppress them. Orthodox medicine, on the other hand, regards symptoms more as a manifestation of the disease, which are to be opposed or suppressed rather than supported.

fever

cough

pain

Homeopathy views a symptom such as pain, fever, or a cough as an expression of the disease and something to be encouraged rather than suppressed. Encouraging symptoms in this way helps to give the immune system a boost and stimulates the body to heal itself.

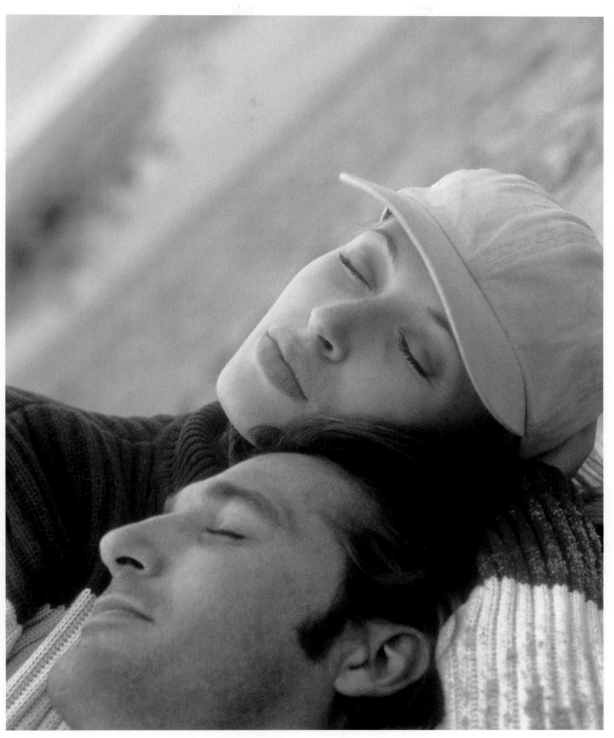

Homeopaths take into account physical, mental, and
emotional factors, including physical appearance,
personality, and temperament, before making a
diagnosis and prescribing a remedy.

The **origins** of **homeopathy**

MERCURY

Hahnemann came to his simple but revolutionary idea about like curing like by noticing that some common illnesses of his time seemed to be best treated by drugs that produced similar symptoms to those produced by the original disease. Intermittent fever (malaria), for example, could be treated, to some degree, with a newly discovered drug of the period, Peruvian bark or cinchona, from which quinine is derived, while syphilis could be controlled by the use of mercury. Both of these drugs brought about similar symptoms to those of the diseases they seemed to help cure.

Hahnemann was excited by this observation and began to draw in his students, friends, and family to test many other contemporary drugs. He hoped to discover what symptoms they could cause in healthy people, and hence, what they could cure in sick people. The tests he conducted were called "provings," from the German *prüfung* meaning "experiment." Over time, his supporters, called "provers," took repeated doses of substances already used in the medicine of his day, such as aconite, arsenic, belladonna, and silver nitrate, and by this method established the range of symptoms that each substance might cause and therefore cure. The provers took the drugs over a long period of time. As they did so, they carefully recorded all the effects of the substances: psychological, emotional, and physical. These detailed descriptions formed the basis of the first collections of symptom profiles, or pictures, of remedies, collectively called *Materia Medica*. These pictures of remedies are still used today, although now they have been vastly expanded by further "provings" and information that have been acquired over two hundred years of clinical experience.

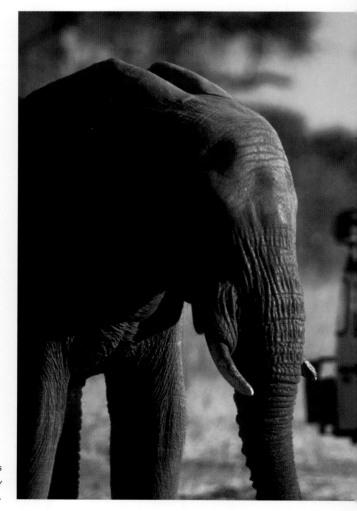

One of the first remedies Hahnemann studied was Peruvian Bark. From this mineral he produced the remedy China, which is still used today by many travelers.

THE VITAL FORCE

What Hahnemann had discovered was a method of making use of the self-healing power of the body. Nowadays, we in the West call this the immune system or the immune and defense system. Hahnemann called it the "vital force," an energetic force inherent in the body, which could be compared with the energy force of Chinese medicine known as *chi*. Homeopathy seeks to cooperate with and strengthen this energy, the vital force, in order to encourage the body to heal itself.

The energy that Hahnemann called vital force can be found in the teachings of other cultures too. Indian yogis, for example, call this invisible energy *prana*, and the Japanese call it *ki*.

The homeopath's aim is therefore to strengthen the vital force, or the immune system, so that it can resist harmful germs and viruses. The homeopath also believes that all parts of the body are interrelated and therefore treats the whole person, rather than concentrating only on the part of the body that is diseased.

CHI

The energy that Hahnemann described as the "vital force" is similar to the invisible life force that Chinese medical practitioners and sages call *chi*. Chi is believed to be essential for good health.

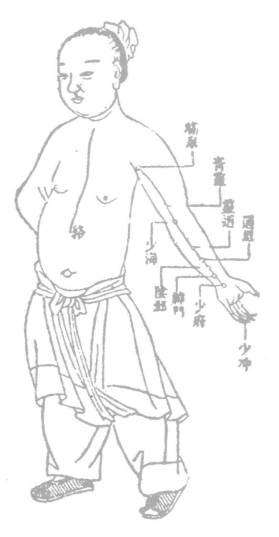

The **development** of **homeopathy**

Dr Hahnemann investigated nearly 200 substances before he died and used them all as remedies in his medical practice. Since then, many more substances have been tested and used as medicines, and now there are more than 3,000 homeopathic medicines available.

Early homeopathic remedies came main[ly] from plants and metals, but Hahnemann later added substances from other sources: these included minerals and chemicals, and creatures such as the bumble bee and the cuttlefish.

EARLY EXPERIMENTS

In the early days of homeopathy, most remedies were made from the plants and metals that had been used regularly in the orthodox medicine of that time, such as chamomilla, pulsatilla, mercury, magnesium, and nitric acid. However, Hahnemann was quick to see the healing potential in other substances that conventional medicine did not use. For instance, he decided to test sepia, a brown, inky liquid put out by squids and cuttlefish to conceal themselves from predators. Artists used it as a paint, and when one of Hahnemann's painter friends became severely depressed, the homeopath wondered whether his friend's habit of sucking his brushes while painting might have been responsible for the condition. After testing sepia, he found that it could indeed cause depression in a person. From this observation, Hahnemann developed a remedy that has proved invaluable for treating people who are overwhelmed by depression, or who suffer from apathy, frustration, irritability, and exhaustion.

CUTTLEFISH

FAR LEFT *Hahnemann tested sepia, the cuttlefish ink used as a paint by artists, and found that it could cause depression in people.*

LATER RESEARCH

Since Hahnemann's time, many other substances have been brought into use as remedies, including exotic plants, trees, minerals, metals, modern drugs, and even

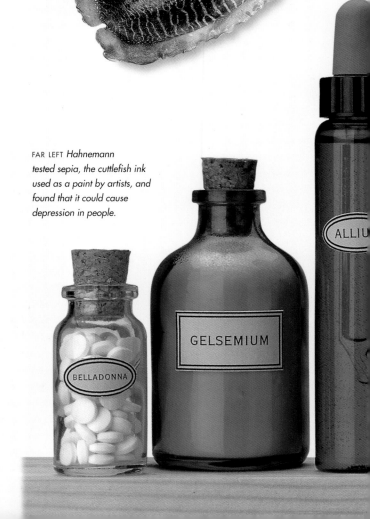

BELLADONNA

GELSEMIUM

ALLIU[M]

disease substances themselves. In fact, any substance whatever can be turned into a homeopathic remedy, provided we know what symptoms it can cause and therefore what it can cure. All the remedies are tested in the same ways as those originally devised by Hahnemann: a symptom picture is built up first, both from the provings and then, over time, from the clinical experience of using the remedies in real medical situations to cure people.

None of the substances used in homeopathy are tested on animals. Since all the symptom pictures are based on a study of the effects of substances on people, they include a great deal of evidence about the psychological and emotional effects of the substances. The provers noted such things as: pains feeling like ants crawling over them, or like splinters in them; feelings of panic or despair; a desire to laugh or cry for no reason; changes in their body temperatures, in their food preferences, in their moods; and dreams and preoccupations. Details of this kind help to build up a picture of the remedy. In this way, the homeopath always treats the person, not the disease.

PULSATILLA

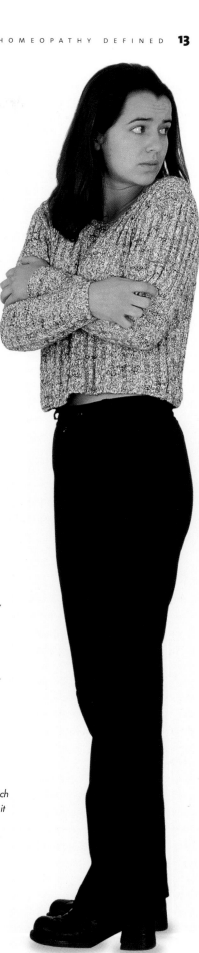

Pulsatilla is an important remedy for women's complaints such as menstrual and menopausal problems, especially when they are characterized by a marked sensitivity to cold and a need for comfort and reassurance.

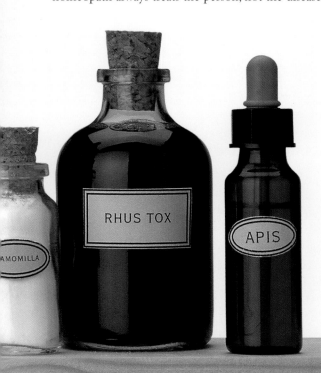

Any substance can become a homeopathic remedy, because each substance can cure the symptoms it causes. The Apis remedy, for example, is made from the honey bee—including its sting—and is used to treat insect stings.

What is a **remedy?**

Each time homeopathic remedies are diluted, they are said to become more potent. You can buy them in tablet, granule, and powder form.

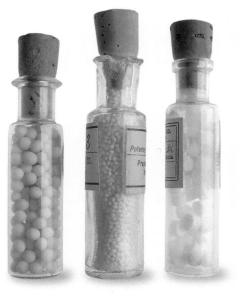

When Hahnemann began practicing homeopathy, he was concerned only with finding the remedy picture most similar to the symptoms of the patient he was treating, and therefore he prescribed substances capable of causing symptoms similar to those of the disease itself. However, he soon found that, when he gave such substances to a patient, he had to give a diluted dose in order to avoid making the patient even more ill by overloading the patient's system with symptoms of both disease and drug.

Homeopaths believe that some energy is released during remedy preparation.

POTENTIZED REMEDIES

In order to avoid overloading patients' systems, Hahnemann began to dilute the medicines gradually. He tried to find the smallest dose that would be curative. He found that the weaker diluted doses not only had a less damaging impact on the patient, but also seemed to be more effective in bringing about a cure. Encouraged by this observation, Hahnemann continued to experiment. He discovered that the diluted medicines became even more effective if they were not only diluted but also shaken up vigorously ("succussed") during dilution.

At that time, Hahnemann believed that the increase in the medicines' power arose because he had released some of the substance's spirit or "vital force." However, modern homeopaths believe that what is released is some of the energy of the substance. The process and its effects are still far from being fully understood, but it is important to remember that the action of a homeopathic remedy is, in some way, energetic and dynamic, rather than chemical or herbal.

DILUTION AND POTENCIES

Nowadays, in order to convert the original substances into potentized, or dynamized, remedies, the homeopathic pharmacist puts a small amount of the medicinal substance into a vial (in a soluble form), adds 99 parts of water and a touch of alcohol, and shakes the solution. This is known as the first "potency" and is termed "1c." A drop is then taken from this solution, mixed with another 99 parts of water and a touch of alcohol, and shaken to give a potency called "2c." This process is repeated over and over again to give potencies 3c, 4c, 5c, 6c, and so on. The more a remedy is diluted and shaken in this way, the more it is potentized, and the more deeply it acts. The lower, less diluted, potencies are in fact less powerful than the higher ones.

Homeopathic remedies are normally sold in many different potencies ranging from 6c to 100,000c (CM). The most commonly available and widely used of the lower potencies in the US are 6c and 30c. Remedies in the sixth potency are readily available from many chemists and health food shops, and some 30c potency remedies are available from these shops.

In addition, any remedy in any potency can be ordered from the homeopathic pharmacies listed at the back of this book (see page 95). However, the higher potencies should be used only by professional homeopaths. In mainland Europe, where a slightly different way of prescribing remedies is current, pharmacists sell potencies numbered in a slightly different way. However, if you need to buy remedies while you are abroad, you can use them in the same way as the similar English potencies.

With most remedies and in most conditions, it is probably a good idea to start with the 6c potency and move up to the 30c if needed. If a more gradual increase in potency is required, you can dissolve a 6c potency in a glass of water and sip from the glass over time, stirring vigorously between each sip. You can increase the potency very gradually in this way.

Remedies can be produced in many forms: tablets are the most common and convenient, but liquids and granules are also available. The tablets are usually small and sweet, and are quite popular with children.

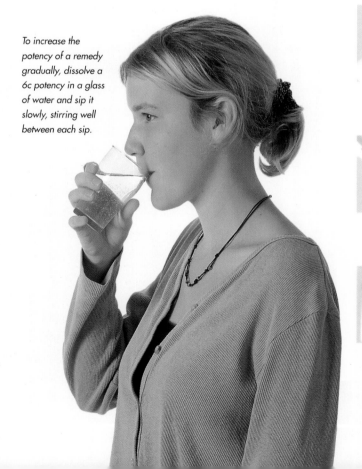

To increase the potency of a remedy gradually, dissolve a 6c potency in a glass of water and sip it slowly, stirring well between each sip.

REMEDY DILUTION

Any substance used to make a homeopathic remedy must be diluted in a solution and successed. This process is called potentization. The more a solution is potentized, the more powerful it becomes.

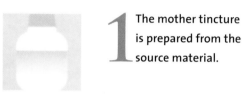

1 The mother tincture is prepared from the source material.

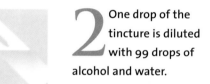

2 One drop of the tincture is diluted with 99 drops of alcohol and water.

3 The remedy is then successed. This makes the 1c potency.

4 Using the 1c potency, the process is then repeated to reach the required potency.

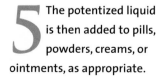

5 The potentized liquid is then added to pills, powders, creams, or ointments, as appropriate.

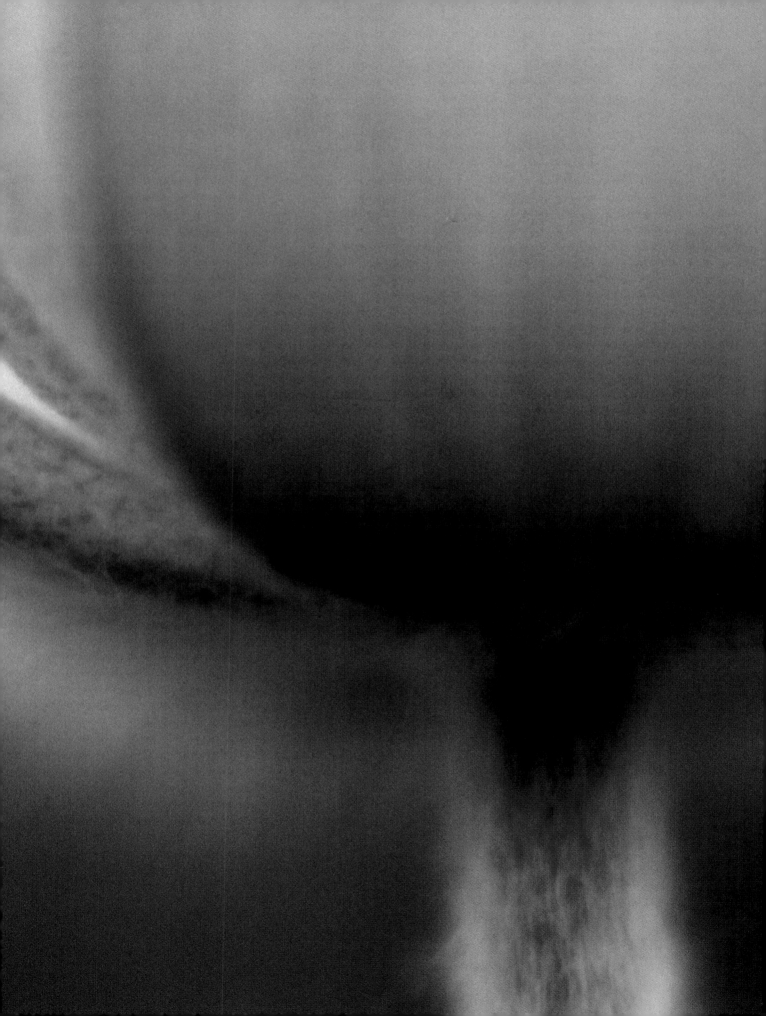

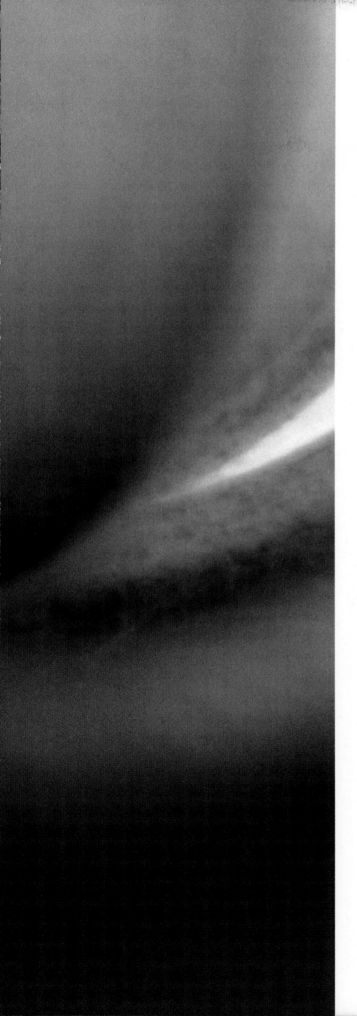

Principles and practice

Homeopathy works on the central concept of treating the whole person. Working on both the emotional and physical levels, remedies are adapted to each patient in order to return the individual to a state of well-being.

Understanding symptoms and remedies

Many different kinds of remedy pictures, or *Materia Medica*, have been developed over the years. Some emphasize physical symptoms, some emphasize psychological symptoms, and others emphasize key, characteristic symptoms. All have something to offer.

Although arsenic is poisonous, it actually makes a good remedy for food poisoning.

The *Materia Medica* in this book includes 30 remedy pictures that are commonly used in homeopathy. They are necessarily brief, but they do give a good general picture, which includes many of the symptoms characteristic of or special to each remedy. As you read the remedy pictures, try to conjure up in your mind what the person described in the picture might look and behave like. How would you react to him or her? How would that person be likely to be ill?

If you try to absorb all the details of a remedy at once, you will sink without trace under a mass of detail, so just try to grasp the main characteristics or individualizing qualities of each remedy, and then you will find it easier. For example, it is easy to tell the difference between a blackbird and a robin, even if we know very little about birds, because we know what is characteristic of them, what is distinctive about them: the black feathers and yellow beak of the blackbird clearly distinguish it from a robin, with its brown feathers and red breast. We need not bother with the finer details: the main features speak for themselves. It is the same with remedies.

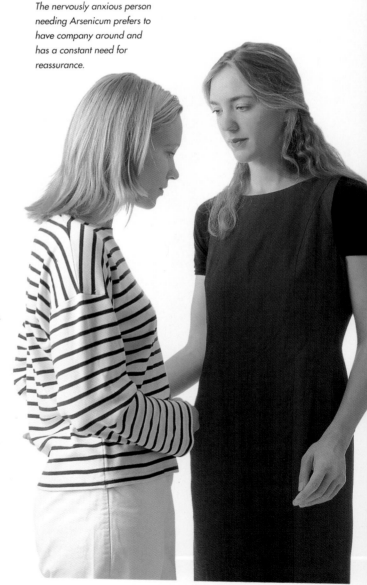

The nervously anxious person needing Arsenicum prefers to have company around and has a constant need for reassurance.

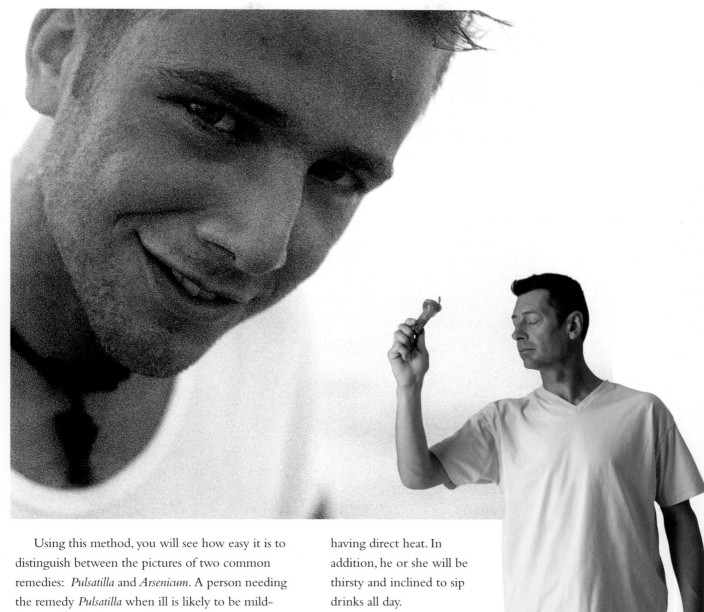

Using this method, you will see how easy it is to distinguish between the pictures of two common remedies: *Pulsatilla* and *Arsenicum*. A person needing the remedy *Pulsatilla* when ill is likely to be mild-tempered, weepy, and clingy, and to feel better if there are people around for company and conversation. He or she is likely to be generally chilly yet uncomfortable in a warm room, and can be badly affected by heat. When ill, this person will be thirstless.

A person needing *Arsenicum* will also feel better if there are people around to talk to, but he or she will not be so tearful. A person needing *Arsenicum* will be more nervously anxious than a person needing *Pulsatilla*, and more critical. This person is also chilly, but will feel better for being in a warm room or having direct heat. In addition, he or she will be thirsty and inclined to sip drinks all day.

The symptoms highlighted here are some of the individualizing characteristics that can help you distinguish between these two remedies. Just as a bird with a red breast cannot be an English blackbird, *Pulsatilla* cannot be comfortable in a warm room and *Arsenicum* cannot be happy alone when ill.

ABOVE *Pulsatilla types feel worse in warm, stuffy atmospheres, but better for cool, fresh air.*

TOP *People needing Arsenicum feel better for warmth and movement.*

The **complete** picture

Complete pictures of remedies include a wide range of so-called "symptoms." Some might clearly be symptoms of illness: for example, difficulty breathing, pain in the right side, and heavy bleeding. However, some seem to be scarcely more than character traits: for example, bad temper in the morning, reserved, weepy, introverted, untidy, and critical. Others may seem to be simply descriptions of physical appearance: for example, red-faced, pale-skinned, or furrowed brow.

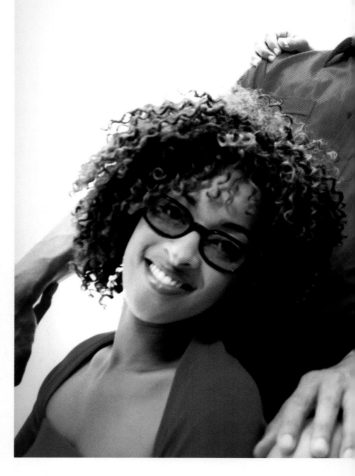

CONSTITUTIONAL TYPES

Homeopaths consider that each person has a basic way of being, in both health and in disease, and that this way of being may sometimes be reflected in a single homeopathic remedy picture. When we classify a person's state in this way, we call it his or her constitutional picture or type. When a person is ill, some of these characteristics may become clearer and more obvious, but they will be only exaggerations or extensions of the normal way of being of that person. These are some of the most valuable symptoms to spot.

A *Pulsatilla* constitutional type, therefore, would be generally mild-mannered, sociable, pleasant, easily emotional, chilly, and thirstless, whether that person was ill or not. If that person is ill, these features would still be part of his or her picture, but one or more of them might be exaggerated or distorted. The person might become more emotional or more chilly, for instance, or might develop catarrh and related symptoms more readily than other types. He or she would be inclined to feel nauseous after eating fatty foods and have poor circulation and trouble with veins. All these would be the kinds of ill health commonly suffered by a person of the *Pulsatilla* type.

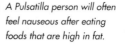

A Pulsatilla person will often feel nauseous after eating foods that are high in fat.

when they are acutely ill. In addition, a person may find his or her own constitutional remedy to be helpful when ill, or may become temporarily sensitive to another polychrest remedy. It is when the remedy matches both states that it acts most deeply.

It is sometimes assumed that a person will display the features of only one constitutional picture throughout life: however, this is very rarely the case. Most people tend to conform to the pictures of a few closely related remedies at various times during their lives. Children usually have simpler constitutional pictures and it is often easier to prescribe a single remedy for them.

When choosing a remedy for someone, that person's healthy characteristics are often as important as the symptoms of the illness. The way the patient is when healthy can be as important as the way the person is when ill.

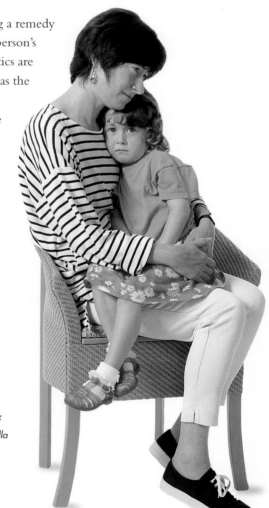

In homeopathy, it is important to study the way people are when they are healthy as well as how they behave when they are ill.

A person's general way of being might conform to this remedy picture in health and in disease; on the other hand, he or she might fit a particular remedy picture only when suffering from an acute illness. Children, for instance, can have many different constitutions, but most of them tend to need *Pulsatilla*

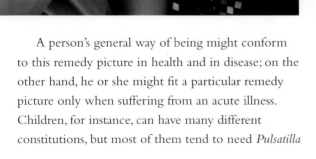

Like adults, children can have many different constitutions, but many of them tend to need Pulsatilla when they are acutely ill.

Types of **illness**

As far as treatment is concerned, this book is mainly about acute (brief) and minor illnesses. Homeopathy can also treat major and chronic (long-lasting) illnesses, but the treatment of these complaints should be undertaken only by a qualified homeopath. If, in the course of using this book, you see indications of serious illness, then please consult a homeopath. Many people also consult homeopaths when they are well: they have treatment for their constitutional state, and keep themselves in balance, rather than waiting until they are seriously ill.

Use homeopathic remedies for minor ailments such as colds, but for serious illnesses see a homeopath.

ACUTE AND CHRONIC CONDITIONS

Acute illnesses come and go of their own accord. Some can be serious and may be life-threatening: some fevers or influenza, for example. Most acute illnesses are less dangerous but still painful, such as fear, anxiety, coughs, colds, cystitis, earache, headache, and migraine. Chronic conditions do not normally get better by themselves and will just get steadily worse unless there is medical intervention. These conditions vary in kind: some may be life-threatening in acute episodes, such as asthma or colitis; others, such as persistent catarrh, repeated thrush, or piles, are not so serious in themselves but may indicate the presence of a deeper disorder that needs to be addressed. Other conditions, such as eczema, arthritis, or psoriasis, are not immediately life-threatening but can cause a great deal of pain and distress and do not usually get better unless treated.

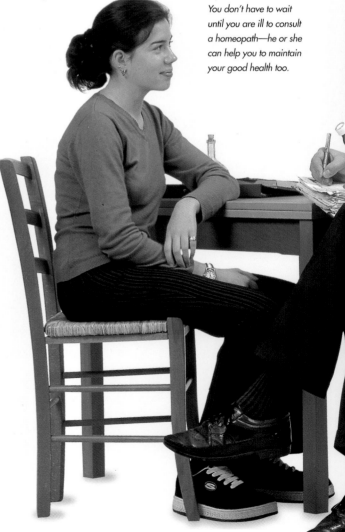

You don't have to wait until you are ill to consult a homeopath—he or she can help you to maintain your good health too.

The purpose of this book is to make clear the basic principles of homeopathy so that you can feel confident about treating yourself for acute conditions and have an informed understanding of the treatment a professional homeopath is likely to prescribe for chronic conditions. You will also develop a knowledge of the kinds of symptoms that are useful to a professional homeopath.

Since homeopathy relies on matching the observable symptoms of the patient when ill to the observable symptoms of the remedy picture, remedies can be prescribed safely in cases of acute or minor illness in the way outlined in this book. To prescribe successfully in a case of chronic disease, however, a much greater understanding of the total disease process is needed and you should always consult a homeopath first.

Homeopathy is very effective for treating a wide range of ailments, from minor complaints to chronic illnesses.

headache
fear
persistent catarrh
coughs
asthma
migraine
anxiety
earache
colds
piles
colitis
arthritis
repeated thrush
cystitis
psoriasis
eczema

No two people are the same, so it is important to build up an accurate remedy picture of the patient before choosing a remedy. If you are in any doubt or the symptoms persist, consult a homeopath.

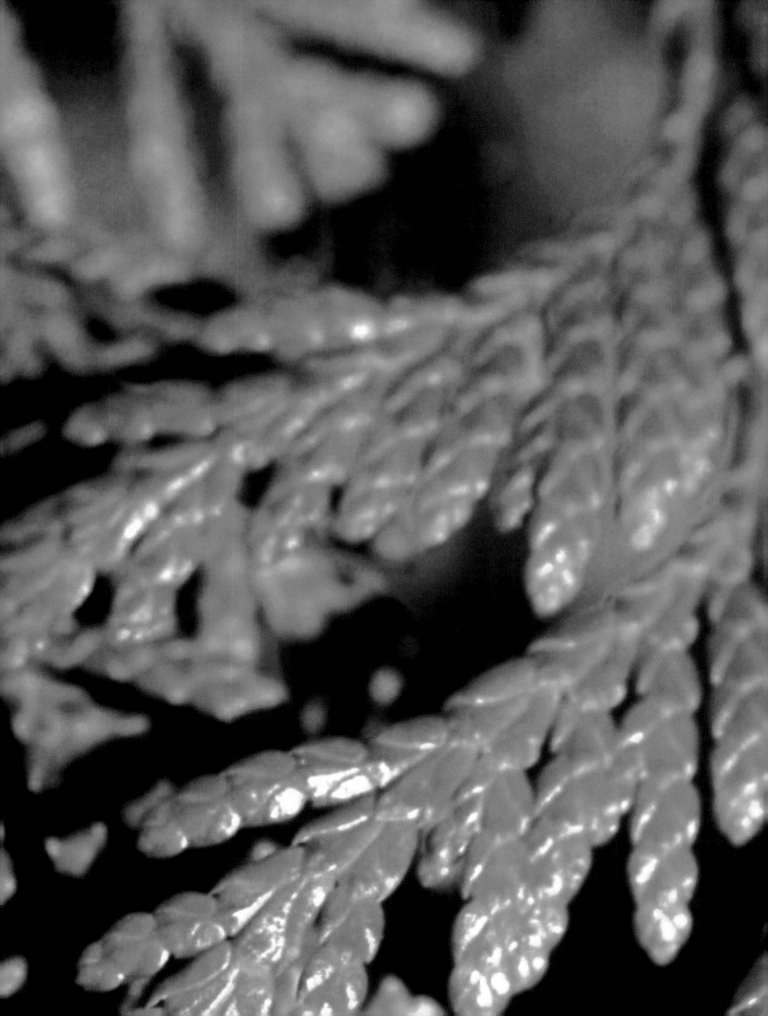

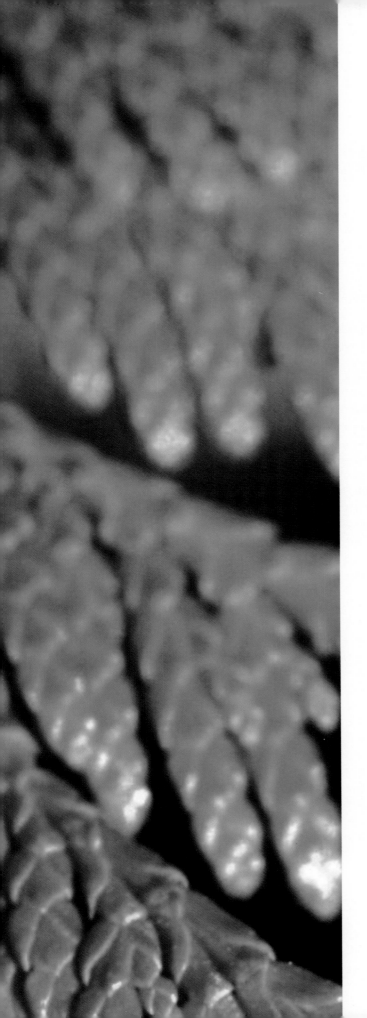

Homeopathy
in action

In this section, we cover how to identify symptoms and find the appropriate remedy. Homeopathy is as good as your ability to choose the right remedy. This involves carefully distinguishing between remedy pictures and learning to study the whole constitution of the patient, in order to successfully match the two.

Identifying
symptoms

It will be obvious by now that a homeopathic symptom picture encompasses more features of the patient than orthodox medicine normally associates with disease. A homeopathic symptom picture attempts to identify everything that is taking place within the patient at the time of the illness. All these things are regarded as symptoms expressing a single mind-body condition. Everything about the patient may be a clue to the remedy.

Look for any significant changes or symptoms that have become exaggerated since their onset, such as marked changes in appetite.

CHOOSING A REMEDY

To demonstrate how to go about choosing a remedy, let us take earache as an example. Ear pain itself could suggest several remedies. From the remedies that we are considering in this book, *Aconite, Belladonna, Chamomilla, Hepar sulf., Merc. sol, Pulsatilla, Silica,* and *Sulfur* are all remedies that include pain in the ear as an important part of their symptom picture. From here, we need to find further details, more particular, characterizing factors. For example, is the person with earache weepy or irritable? Chilly or hot? Red-faced or pale? Is the person hungry, or has he or she gone off food? Anything that has changed or become exaggerated in the patient since the pain started will be useful to notice. These symptoms will undoubtedly point to different remedies, even though many remedy pictures include earache.

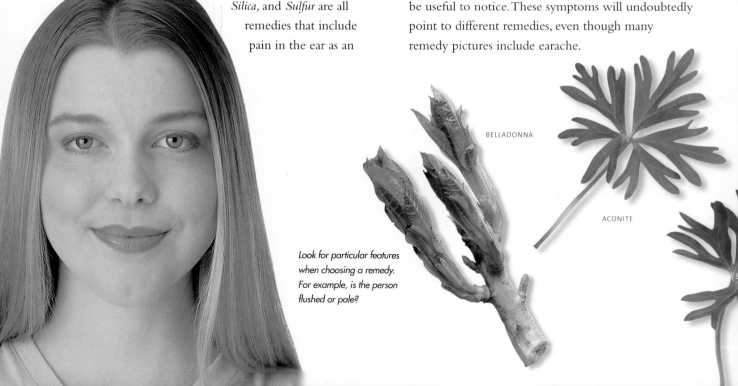

BELLADONNA

ACONITE

Look for particular features when choosing a remedy. For example, is the person flushed or pale?

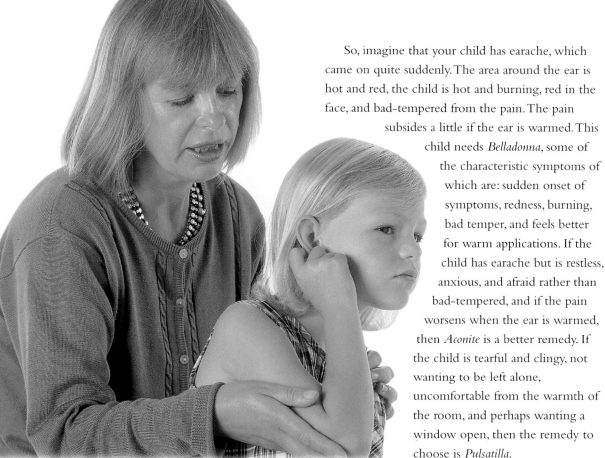

So, imagine that your child has earache, which came on quite suddenly. The area around the ear is hot and red, the child is hot and burning, red in the face, and bad-tempered from the pain. The pain subsides a little if the ear is warmed. This child needs *Belladonna*, some of the characteristic symptoms of which are: sudden onset of symptoms, redness, burning, bad temper, and feels better for warm applications. If the child has earache but is restless, anxious, and afraid rather than bad-tempered, and if the pain worsens when the ear is warmed, then *Aconite* is a better remedy. If the child is tearful and clingy, not wanting to be left alone, uncomfortable from the warmth of the room, and perhaps wanting a window open, then the remedy to choose is *Pulsatilla*.

No two children with earache are the same: if the child is bad-tempered and warmth eases the pain, try Belladonna, but if the child is afraid and the pain worsens for warmth, try Aconite instead.

The remedy Hepar sulf. is prepared chemically by heating together ground sulfur and powdered oyster shell.

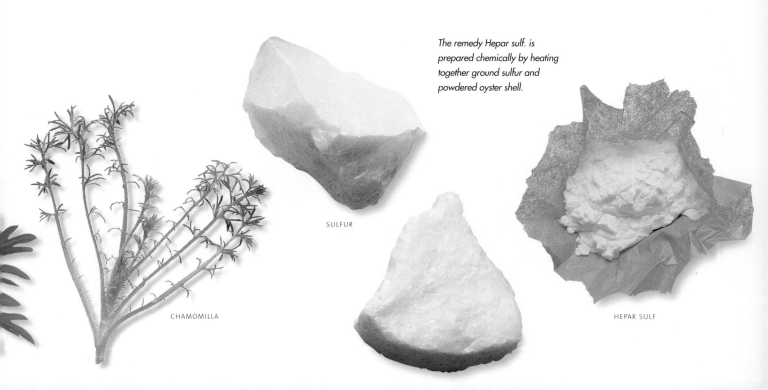

CHAMOMILLA

SULFUR

HEPAR SULF

TREATING THE PERSON, NOT THE ILLNESS

If your child does not have earache after all, but instead has a cold or measles, and is hot, red in the face, and bad-tempered, the remedy is still *Belladonna;* in the same way, if the child is tearful and clingy, not wanting to be left alone, and uncomfortable from the warmth of the room, the remedy is still *Pulsatilla.*

This is one of the hardest principles to grasp about homeopathy, but once you have grasped it everything becomes simpler. Since you are treating the *person* and not the disease, the remedy for the person may remain the same, even though the illness is apparently different. The important symptoms are those that tell you how the *person* is feeling and behaving when ill, while the actual name of the illness is very low in importance on the list.

So we need to ask, is the person ill in a *Belladonna* way or a *Pulsatilla* way? What helps us to choose the right remedy is the distinctive way in which the patient reacts to the illness, in the whole of his or her person and personality: for example, through feelings, behavior, body temperature, and appetite. Look at the bigger picture, for as complete a picture as possible.

Though this process gets more complicated in chronic illness, the principle is always the same: try to match as much as possible of the patient's picture in illness to a remedy picture. Put more emphasis on the general state of the patient than on the particular illness from which he or she is suffering. Look for the marked characteristics of the patient when ill and match them to the marked characteristics of the remedies described in the *Materia Medica.*

Usually, emotional and psychological symptoms, and general physical symptoms, such as temperature preferences and food cravings, give a better indication of the remedy than particular symptoms of the illness itself, but try to make sure the remedy picture you choose includes any important particular symptoms of the illness in order to get a complete picture.

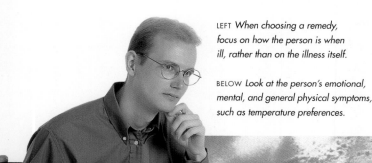

LEFT *When choosing a remedy, focus on how the person is when ill, rather than on the illness itself.*

BELOW *Look at the person's emotional, mental, and general physical symptoms, such as temperature preferences.*

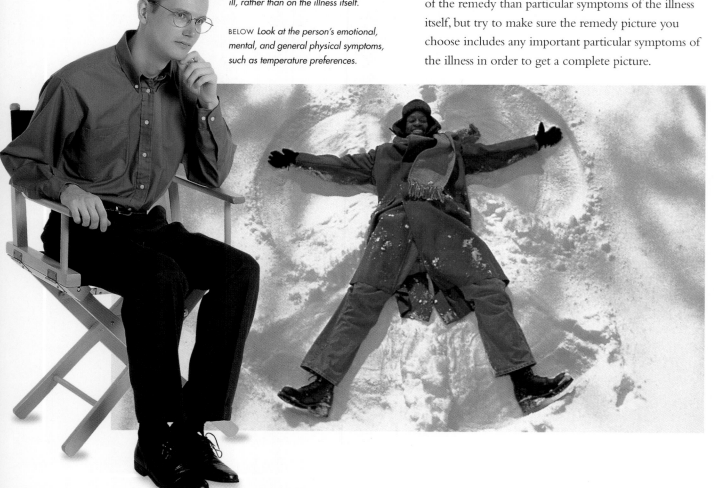

PSYCHOLOGICAL SYMPTOMS

The psychological/emotional picture is extremely important in homeopathy. It frequently gives the strongest indications for the remedy, even when the illness seems to be entirely physical. It helps to pinpoint the condition and characterize it. In acute illness, the psychological response can often show itself in what appears to be a complete change of character—the patient is "not himself," we might say. At other times, the patient may indeed be himself, but more so. For instance, a person who is normally quite shy and reserved will become almost reclusive, so that what had been just a character trait becomes overemphasized to the point of disability. Either of these types of change is an important symptom and should be noted.

In chronic illness too, a habitual mode of being, or a long-established personality pattern, can be just as much of a symptom as is long-standing joint pain, how someone's digestion works, or the nature of his or her skin. So it is important to ask questions, in order to build up a complete picture. What is his or her mood usually like? Irritable? Tearful? Cheerful despite the pain? Does the person want company or to be alone? How does the person's mood appear now: quieter than usual or more talkative?

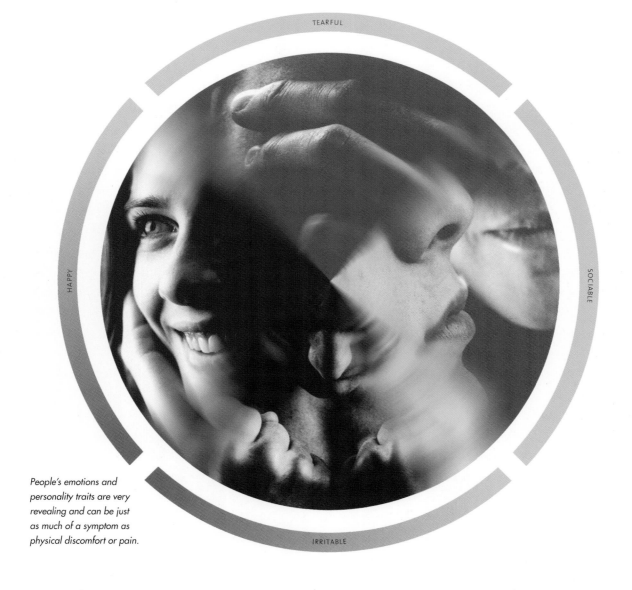

TEARFUL

HAPPY

SOCIABLE

IRRITABLE

People's emotions and personality traits are very revealing and can be just as much of a symptom as physical discomfort or pain.

GENERAL PHYSICAL SYMPTOMS

General physical symptoms, states, or changes are very important because they affect the whole person.

How is the patient feeling physically? Hot, chilly, sweaty, dry, thirsty, thirstless? Is he or she unusually hungry, off food, craving certain foods, disliking others? Over-sensitive to pain or not feeling it as much as you would expect? Droopy and exhausted, or full of frantic energy? Things that make the person as a whole feel better or worse are very useful clues to the remedy: for example, is the person better or worse for heat, cold, damp, warmth, fresh air, stuffy rooms, winter, summer, night, morning, day, evening, ice cream, butter?

These general physical symptoms, like the psychological ones, may change during the course of disease or may become exaggerated. They are more important for choosing the right remedy than looking at particular symptoms of the complaint itself.

PARTICULAR SYMPTOMS

These will usually include the symptoms of the actual illness or complaint. As such, they often affect a particular part of the person. For example, earache, period pain, colds, and joint pain can all be localized within one part or system of the patient's body. In homeopathy, these symptoms are less important clues to the remedy than the general physical symptoms just described, because particular symptoms are usually not very individual. They relate more to the

General physical symptoms can be useful clues when choosing a remedy, so look at how a person feels in different temperatures, at different times of day, and when eating and drinking certain things.

MORNING

COLDS

SUMMER

NIGHT

WINTER

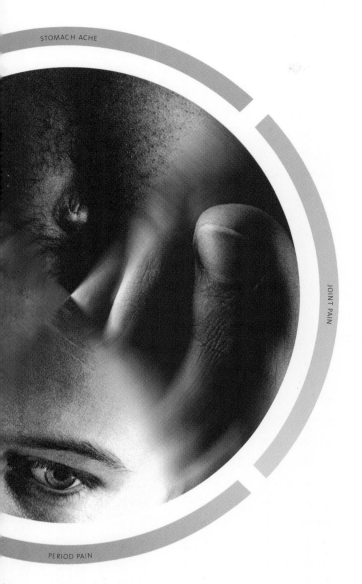

STOMACH ACHE

JOINT PAIN

PERIOD PAIN

*Particular symptoms of the illness
are usually localized to certain
parts of the body, such as earache,
period pain, or joint pain, and are
not in themselves helpful unless
they are unusual in some way.*

LOOKING FOR THE UNUSUAL

When you are looking for a suitable remedy, remember that the more unusual a particular symptom is in connection with the complaint, the more important it becomes. It is not unusual for a cold to be accompanied by a cough, but if the cough has markedly different characteristics from the usual ones associated with that complaint, a more precise description of the nature of the cough would be helpful. For example, the person affected might feel as if he or she has a splinter in the throat (a clue for *Hepar sulf.*), or might hold the ribs when coughing because the movement will hurt (a clue for *Bryonia*).

These apparently small distinguishing features in every sick person are the important clues, the things that mark the cold as this particular person's cold, not just any cold. No two colds are quite the same. The nearer you get to establishing what is different or distinctive, what is individual about the condition in a particular person, the nearer you are to finding the remedy that will relieve it.

In forming a picture of a patient, the homeopath will not just rely on what the patient says, but will also notice *how* the patient says it, whether he or she is reserved and uncommunicative about their symptoms (*Natrum mur., Kali carb.*), whether the person is outgoing and helpful (*Phosphorus*), irritable and impatient (*Arsenicum, Nux vomica*), or sceptical but interested, asking questions, for instance, about how homeopathy works (*Sulfur*), or extremely anxious about the illness (*Arsenicum*). The homeopath will also note other things, such as color and nature of the skin. Extreme pallor might indicate *China*, redness *Sulfur*, blueish-purple *Lachesis*. Has the person got a particular smell? Sourness might indicate *Calc. carb.*, for example, or old cheese might indicate *Hepar sulf.* All these observations provide valuable clues.

disease itself than to the person. Particular symptoms of the illness are really only of interest when they deviate from what might have been expected of that named illness or when they combine with other symptoms in an unusual or uncharacteristic way, or when they are in some way odd.

So "diarrhea," for example, is a condition with a particular symptom: loose stools. "Diarrhea with headache" makes the symptom a little more useful because not all remedies that might cure diarrhea have diarrhea with headache. "Joint pain" is not a very helpful symptom because it occurs in many remedies. "Joint pain with indigestion" or "with headache" would individualize the condition more.

Finding the remedy

Once you have built up a symptom picture of the person, you need to match it to the right remedy. The easiest way to do this is to look up the particular complaint in the A–Z of common ailments (see pages 72–87). See which remedies are suggested there for the complaint you are treating, and then find those remedies in the *Materia Medica* section (see pages 38–71). Try to identify which remedy best matches the person overall. Remember that you are not looking for an identical match, only for a remedy picture that is *similar* to the patient's total symptom picture. The stronger the similarity between remedy and symptom pictures, the greater the likelihood of a rapid and complete cure.

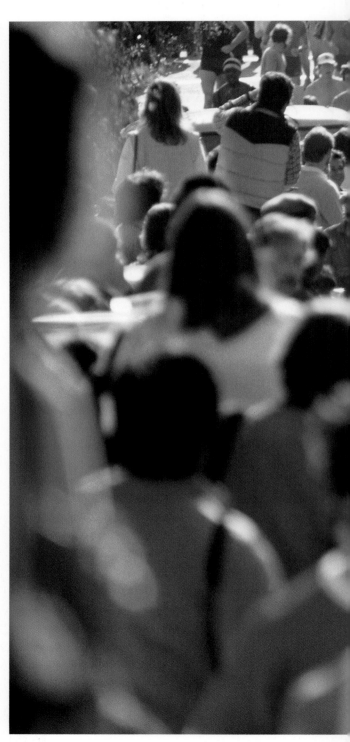

Remember that it is more important to match the psychological/emotional and general physical symptoms than the particular symptoms of the complaint. And remember that what the remedy is doing is stimulating the person's own immune system to a more vigorous response than it is capable of by itself. Once that has been done, the self-healing system can keep going by itself, at least in the type of illness you will be treating. Finally, if you choose the wrong remedy, nothing terrible will happen. Ask more questions, think it over again, then try another remedy. All you will have lost is time.

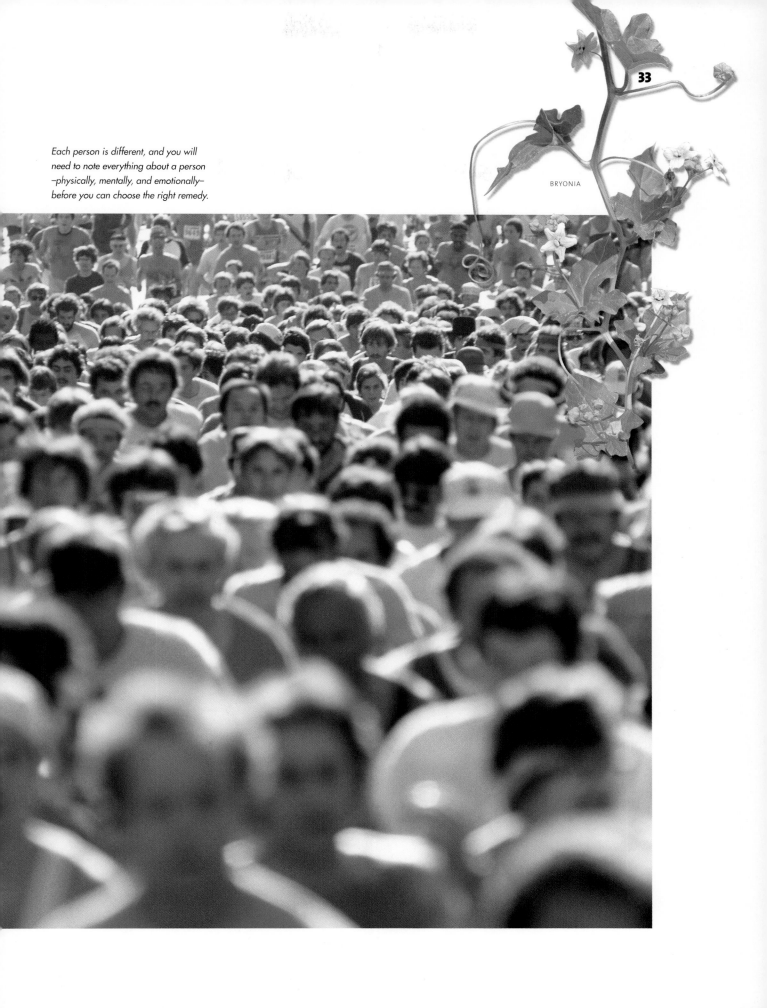

*Each person is different, and you will
need to note everything about a person
–physically, mentally, and emotionally–
before you can choose the right remedy.*

BRYONIA

Giving or taking remedies

The thirty remedies described in this book can mostly be bought over the counter in the 6c potency. If you are making up a kit to keep at home, some remedies, such as *Aconite, Arnica, Belladonna*, and *Chamomilla*, should be bought if possible in the 30c potency. This is because the acute circumstances in which you are likely to use these remedies lend themselves better to the use of a higher potency.

When you have decided what remedy you are going to prescribe and in what potency, give just one dose (one tablet) at a time. Try not to touch it: tip it into the person's mouth either from the cap of the bottle or from a spoon or a clean, folded piece of paper. The person should then suck the tablet for a few minutes, or suck and then chew if the tablet is a hard one; leave 15 minutes before eating or drinking. If you accidentally drop a tablet, you should throw it away. All these precautions are necessary not because it is dangerous to touch the remedies, but merely to protect the medicine from being contaminated by strong smells or tastes and therefore perhaps making it less effective.

If you want homeopathic remedies to work at their best, and if you want to be as clear as possible as to their effects, you should not take other medicines at the same time. However, it is not always possible to be purist about this, and if you want to take them at the same time as other medicines, it is safe to do so. *Never* stop taking a prescribed orthodox medicine without consulting your homeopath or doctor first.

When taking homeopathic remedies, always try to make sure that at least 15 minutes elapse either side without eating or drinking anything.

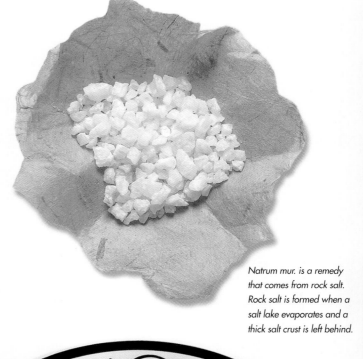

Natrum mur. is a remedy that comes from rock salt. Rock salt is formed when a salt lake evaporates and a thick salt crust is left behind.

To protect a remedy from contamination, do not touch it. Instead, tip it from the bottle onto a clean teaspoon and take at once.

If you have not got a suitable spoon to hand, you can fold a clean piece of paper and use it to tip the remedy into your mouth.

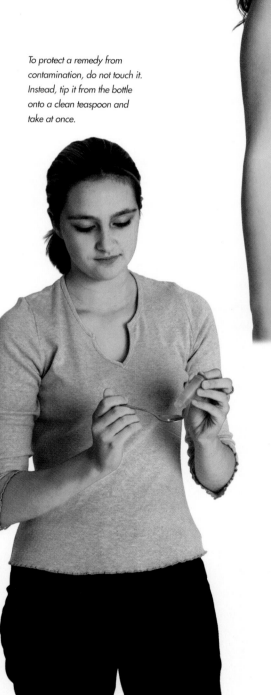

When you are away from home, improvise by tipping the remedy into the bottle cap, then transferring it to your mouth. Don't let the cap touch your lips though.

Waiting for the **remedy** to work

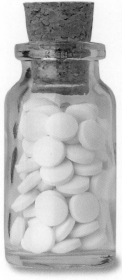

Homeopathic remedies do not take over the body's healing system. Instead, they encourage the body to heal itself.

After giving or taking a remedy, you should wait and watch for a while. You may notice a reaction very quickly, but since you are using low potencies, you may need to repeat the dose several times before any sustained effect will be noticed. If the illness has arisen quickly and developed to a crisis, then you can expect a quick healing reaction after one dose, or after two or three repetitions. If the illness has developed slowly, then the healing reaction is likely to be slower, and you may need to repeat a dose three or four times a day for a few days before noticing any change. Do not be afraid to repeat a dose quickly in an acute illness, yet do not be in too much hurry to repeat a dose in a slower, more long-lasting one. Remember you are merely trying to get the body's healing system to go into action on its own behalf, not to take over from it. So give the remedy just as long as you need to start the self-healing process.

If you are trying to do something like stop a hemorrhage or soothe an attack of colic or an earache, then you should expect quick relief if you have chosen the right remedy. When the body is in crisis, it takes up the remedy very quickly. If you have given the chosen remedy three times within an hour, say, and have observed no effect, then you should reconsider the remedy: if it still seems to be the right one, then try a higher potency. If you do not have the remedy in a higher potency, dissolve a tablet of the sixth potency in a glass of water (preferably sterilized or mineral water), and tell the person to take sips from that, stirring vigorously between each sip. Each sip should be regarded as a separate dose.

When you are increasing the potency of a particular remedy, remember to use pure mineral water or sterilized water for dissolving the tablet. Stir well between each sip and regard each sip as a separate dose.

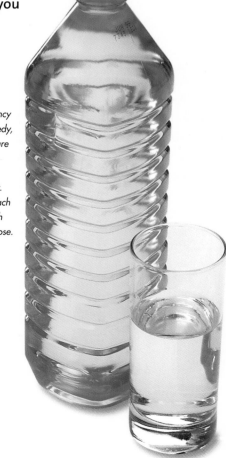

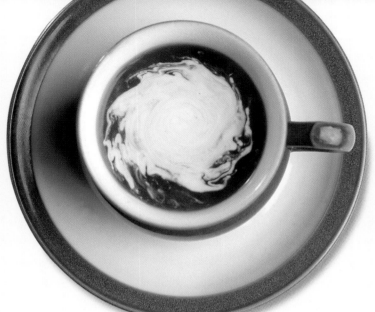

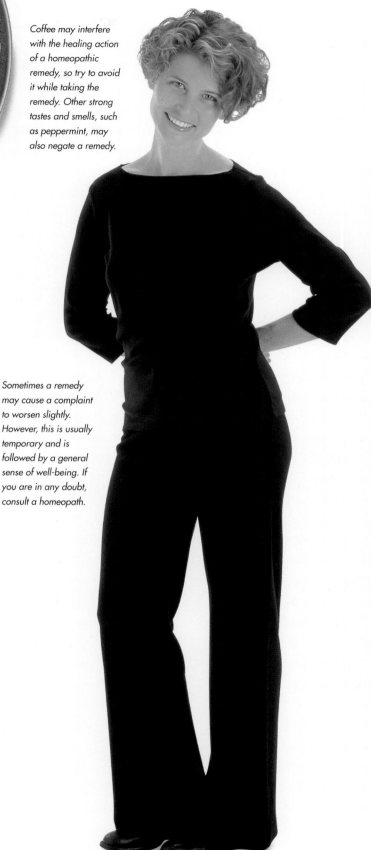

Coffee may interfere with the healing action of a homeopathic remedy, so try to avoid it while taking the remedy. Other strong tastes and smells, such as peppermint, may also negate a remedy.

If, on the other hand, you are giving the remedy for a long-standing and stubborn condition, such as joint pain, you should not necessarily expect results until you have given the remedy for, say, three or four times a day over several days in the 6c potency. If the improvement is slight or uncertain, then repeat the remedy. If there is a clear improvement, then do not repeat the remedy until the improvement seems to have come to a halt.

TEMPORARY SETBACKS

Sometimes the use of homeopathic remedies causes a condition to worsen temporarily before it gets better. This is the aggravation that many people have heard of in connection with homeopathy. It is usually quite slight and short-lasting, and is accompanied or followed by a general sense of well-being, even though a particular symptom may get worse. If there is an aggravation, wait until it has died down before trying the remedy again. If it happens again, then ask a homeopath for advice because this would suggest that the person you are treating is particularly sensitive to the remedy, and there are ways of getting round this.

Sometimes a remedy may cause a complaint to worsen slightly. However, this is usually temporary and is followed by a general sense of well-being. If you are in any doubt, consult a homeopath.

Some homeopaths believe that the action of remedies is interfered with by strong tastes or smells, such as coffee or peppermint. If a remedy you have given does not work, check to see whether the person is accidentally making it inactive by using strong-smelling or strong-tasting substances.

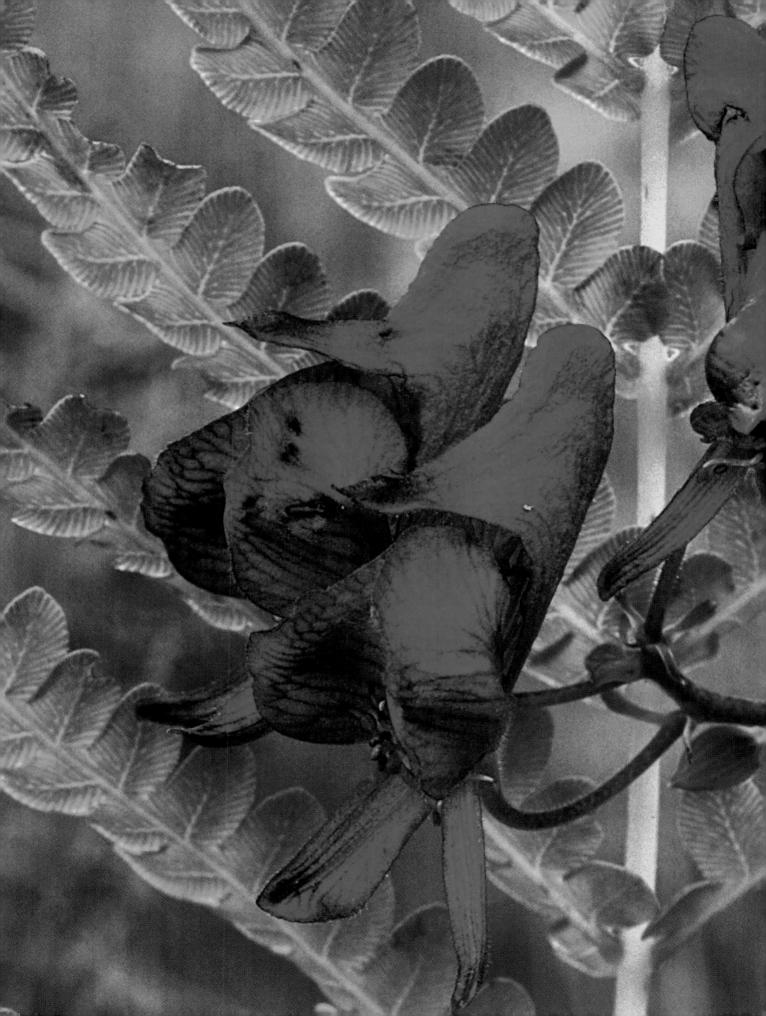

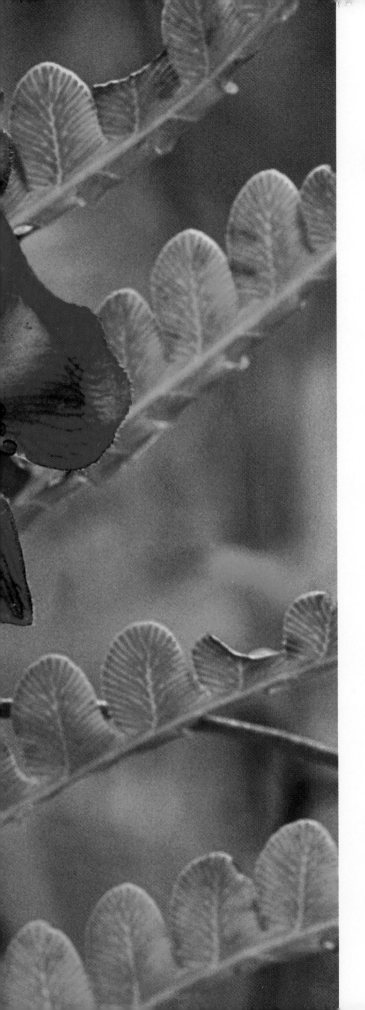

Materia Medica

The *Materia Medica* is a compendium of the principal remedies used in homeopathy. Each remedy is covered in considerable detail to let you choose the one most appropriate for the symptom picture that you wish to treat.

Materia Medica

This *Materia Medica* is a compendium of the most commonly used remedies in homeopathy. Each remedy is described fully—including its chemical derivative, common names and comprehensive details of its remedy profile. This will enable you to find and recognize the precise symptoms you wish to treat. In order to choose the best remedy, first read through the *Materia Medica* in its entirety and familarize yourself with the different choices. As you become more comfortable with the characteristics of the remedies, you will find that you can match these with the constitution of the patient and, in time, will learn the unique personalities of each remedy.

Homeopathy can aid the whole family and the range of remedies in this book will help you treat many everyday ills.

H omeopathic remedy pictures give you information on the many different kinds of minor ailments or more serious illnesses a remedy can treat, as well as describing the specific symptoms involved. The information here will help you to build a complete profile of the patient and remedy by detailing both subjective and physical feelings.

LISTING
The remedies are listed in alphabetical order using the homeopathic name and Latin name.

SYMPTOMS
The "Symptoms" box covers how the patient feels in different environmental situations. One person's symptoms may improve with open air, another's may improve with sleep and warmth.

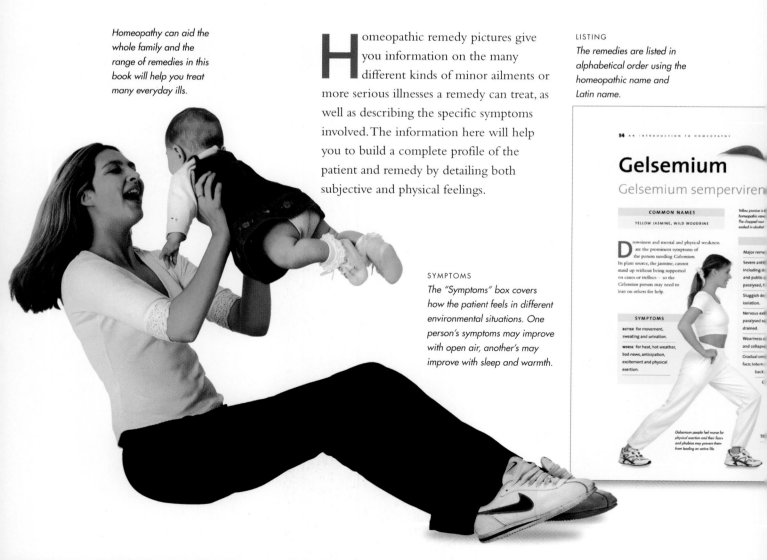

COMMON NAMES

Many of the remedies have common names which may help you familiarize yourself with them.

PROFILE

The remedy profile covers the different characteristics the remedy treats and is essential in diagnosis.

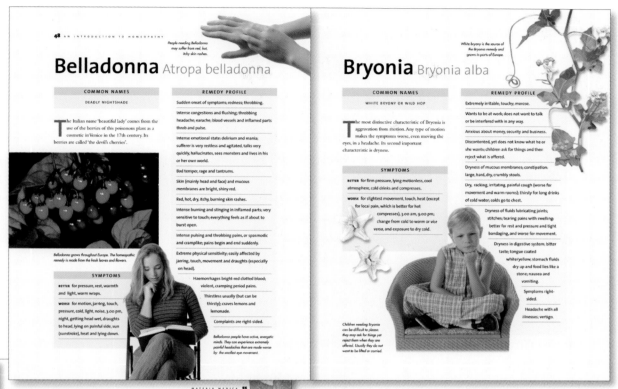

48 AN INTRODUCTION TO HOMEOPATHY

People needing Belladonna may suffer from red, hot, itchy skin rashes.

Belladonna Atropa belladonna

COMMON NAMES	**REMEDY PROFILE**
DEADLY NIGHTSHADE	Sudden onset of symptoms; redness; throbbing.

The Italian name 'beautiful lady' comes from the use of the berries of this poisonous plant as a cosmetic in Venice in the 17th century. Its berries are called 'the devil's cherries'.

Belladonna grows throughout Europe. The homeopathic remedy is made from the fresh leaves and flowers.

REMEDY PROFILE

Intense congestions and flushing; throbbing headache; earache; blood vessels and inflamed parts throb and pulse.

Intense emotional state: delirium and mania; sufferer is very restless and agitated, talks very quickly, hallucinates, sees monsters and lives in his or her own world.

Bad temper, rage and tantrums.

Skin (mainly head and face) and mucous membranes are bright, shiny red.

Red, hot, dry, itchy, burning skin rashes.

Intense burning and stinging in inflamed parts; very sensitive to touch; everything feels as if about to burst open.

Intense pulsing and throbbing pains, or spasmodic and cramplike; pains begin and end suddenly.

Extreme physical sensitivity; easily affected by jarring, touch, movement and draughts (especially on head).

Haemorrhages bright-red clotted blood; violent, cramping period pains.

Thirstless usually (but can be thirsty); craves lemons and lemonade.

Complaints are right-sided.

Belladonna people have active, energetic minds. They can experience extremely painful headaches that are made worse by the smallest eye movement.

SYMPTOMS

BETTER for pressure, rest, warmth and light, warm wraps.

WORSE for motion, jarring, touch, pressure, cold, light, noise, 3.00 pm, night, getting head wet, draughts to head, lying on painful side, sun (sunstroke), heat and lying down.

White bryony is the source of the Bryonia remedy and grows in parts of Europe.

Bryonia Bryonia alba

COMMON NAMES	**REMEDY PROFILE**
WHITE BRYONY OR WILD HOP	Extremely irritable; touchy; morose.

The most distinctive characteristic of Bryonia is aggravation from motion. Any type of motion makes the symptoms worse, even moving the eyes, in a headache. Its second important characteristic is dryness.

SYMPTOMS

BETTER for firm pressure, lying motionless, cool atmosphere, cold drinks and compresses.

WORSE for slightest movement, touch, heat (except for local pain, which is better for hot compresses), 3.00 am, 9.00 pm; change from cold to warm or vice versa, and exposure to dry cold.

Children needing Bryonia can be difficult to please; they may ask for things yet reject them when they are offered. Usually they do not want to be lifted or carried.

REMEDY PROFILE

Wants to be at work; does not want to talk or be interfered with in any way.

Anxious about money, security and business.

Discontented, yet does not know what he or she wants; children ask for things and then reject what is offered.

Dryness of mucous membranes; constipation; large, hard, dry, crumbly stools.

Dry, racking, irritating, painful cough (worse for movement and warm rooms); thirsty for long drinks of cold water; colds go to chest.

Dryness of fluids lubricating joints; stitches; tearing pains with swelling; better for rest and pressure and tight bandaging, and worse for movement.

Dryness in digestive system; bitter taste; tongue coated white/yellow; stomach fluids dry up and food lies like a stone; nausea and vomiting.

Symptoms right-sided.

Headache with all illnesses; vertigo.

COMPARISON

When choosing a remedy or diagnosing a patient, remember to read through all the necessary remedy profiles. The profiles are quite specific, so you should choose one that fits your constitution.

MATERIA MEDICA **55**

Hepar sulph.
Hepar sulphuris calcareum

The Hepar sulph. remedy is also known as calcium sulphide. It is prepared from a mixture of calcium carbonate from oyster shells and powdered sulphur.

COMMON NAMES	**REMEDY PROFILE**
CALCIUM SULPHIDE	Emotionally oversensitive; touchy; irritable, impatient, quarrelsome, angry and abusive.

Hepar sulph's outstanding characteristic is its capacity to respond to and help extreme sensitivity of every sort, to touch, cold, emotion and pain. All troubles and physical symptoms are better for wet weather.

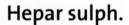

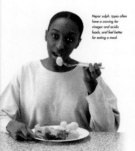

Hepar sulph. types often have a craving for vinegar and acidic foods, and feel better for eating a meal.

REMEDY PROFILE

Hasty and impulsive; ready to burst out.

Impulses to commit suicide.

Physically oversensitive: to touch, surroundings, pain, cold and the least draught.

Infected parts extremely tender to touch: cannot even bear bedclothes.

Slightest pressure causes sharp pain, as if a splinter.

Everything festers and suppurates (gathers or discharges pus); feels sore, as if a boil.

Catarrhal states prominent; catarrhal colds.

Splintering pains in throat or sensation as of a lodged fishbone.

Facial neuralgia; often right-sided after exposure to cold wind.

Thick, cheesy, yellow discharges.

Sour, offensive sweats.

SYMPTOMS

BETTER for eating a meal, staying warm and wrapping up the head.

WORSE for cold, especially dry cold.

PICTURES

Some of the essential characteristics of the remedy or the patient's remedy picture are shown visually.

Aconite Aconitum napellus

COMMON NAMES

MONK'S HOOD, WOLF'S BANE

Aconite symptoms come on suddenly and intensely with anxiety, fear, and restlessness. Intense burning, tingling, shooting pains are characteristic and complaints are often brought on by fright or by being exposed to cold dry weather. The patient has a red, dry, flushed face and burning skin.

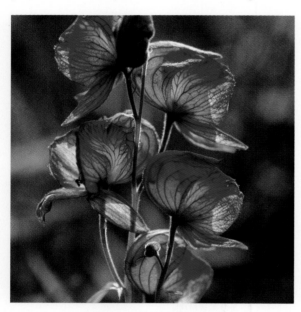

Aconite is a deadly plant that was used as a poison in hunting. It grows wild in mountainous areas of Europe.

SYMPTOMS

BETTER for open air, rest, and perspiration.

WORSE for extreme, sudden cold, cold and dry wind, getting chilled, night (especially midnight), fright, shock, noise, light, and extreme heat.

REMEDY PROFILE

Symptoms come on suddenly, violently, and intensely, like a big storm that blows up quickly and yet soon blows over.

Restlessness and fear: great fear of death; strong sense of when death will happen; fear of crowds, open spaces, going out, and the dark.

Severe anxiety and panic attacks.

Sudden intense, shooting pains; neuralgic pains, especially in the trigeminal area.

Sudden high temperatures, seen in acute feverish illnesses; face is red, dry, and flushed; skin burning; relieved by sweat.

Intense thirst for large quantities of cold water; everything tastes bitter.

Sensitive to light, noise, and touch.

Circulation easily affected: may be sudden flushing, raised blood pressure, hot flushes in menopause, and palpitations.

Use *Aconite* for shock and the effects of shock, even years after the event.

Use *Aconite* for earliest stages of most complaints, initial stages of inflammation, and coughs and earache.

Aconite should be taken at the onset of an infection, especially when the face is red and swollen and there is severe burning pain.

Apis Apis mellifica

The Apis remedy is prepared from the whole honey bee, including its sting, and is very good for easing inflammation.

COMMON NAMES

HONEY BEE

Apis is derived from the sting of a bee and its key symptoms in acute situations are stinging, burning pains or the tight, rosy-skinned watery swellings of a bee sting, whether this is caused by a sore throat, rheumatic inflammation, or the bite or sting of an insect. Bees are restless, move quickly from flower to flower, and are irritable when disturbed. When resting, they can be lazy, indifferent, and apathetic.

The Apis remedy is particularly useful for fever that is accompanied by dry, sensitive skin and a lack of thirst.

SYMPTOMS

BETTER for cold compresses, cold in any form, fresh air, cold bathing, uncovering, change of position, and walking about.

WORSE for heat in any form, stuffy rooms, hot drinks, hot compresses, sleep, touch, pressure, late afternoon (4.00 pm), lying down, fright, rage, vexation, and bad news.

REMEDY PROFILE

Jealousy.

Irritable, fearful, and suspicious.

Depressed apathetic state with a fear of death or of being alone.

Sudden dramatic swelling and inflammation with rosy redness. Watery, puffy swellings, tense and stiff.

Watery swelling around the eyes, eyelids, mouth, face, joints, limbs, or throat (making breathing difficult).

Sudden burning, stinging, sharp pains; pains may wander round body; pains make sufferer cry out.

Urticaria-like eruptions (nettle rash) on the skin with intolerable itching and burning.

High fever where the person is hot, tearful, irritable, sleepy, and delirious; skin is hot, dry, and sweaty by turn. Thirstless.

Body is generally sore and sensitive, worse for touch.

Use *Apis* after a fright, rage, vexation, or bad news.

Watery swellings on the eyelids or the throat may spread to the mouth and make breathing difficult.

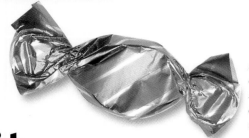

People needing Argent. nit. crave candie, sugar, and sweet foods, but when they eat them they may suffer from diarrhea and sickness.

Argent. nit. Argentum nitricum

COMMON NAMES

SILVER NITRATE

Poisoning with silver nitrate causes great feelings of fear, nervousness, restlessness, and excitability, as well as tremors and twitchings of muscles, poor coordination, and burning sensations. The person's mental faculties become tired and sluggish; they lose ambition.

The Argent. nit. remedy comes from silver nitrate crystals. These crystals are extracted from acanthite (silver ore).

SYMPTOMS

BETTER for cool, fresh air, pressure on the affected part, cold applications, and company.

WORSE for emotion, anxiety, being in closed places, heat, stuffy rooms, eating candies, sugar, intellectual work, emotional stress, night, on waking, before menstruation, and lying on right side.

An Argent. nit. person feels uncomfortable in hot, stuffy rooms and prefers to have cool, fresh air.

REMEDY PROFILE

Impulsive and hurried; feeling driven; tormented by anxious thoughts; wanting to jump from windows and high places.

Extremely nervous of people and crowds; afraid of heights, tall buildings, and open spaces.

Very strong sense of anxious anticipation; always wondering, "what if...?"; worries about health; doubts ability to succeed.

Mentally confused; forgets things easily;

Palpitations and trembling.

Co-ordination difficult; nervous system may be badly affected: neurological conditions such as multiple sclerosis (MS).

Warm-blooded; cannot bear heat; feels claustrophobic in stuffy atmospheres; prone to sudden nervous sweats.

Sensation of a splinter or thorn; pains sharp: they come and go slowly, and tend to be left-sided.

Ulceration of the eyes, stomach, and bowels (ulcerative colitis).

Nervous diarrhea; irritable bowel syndrome; flatulence and wind.

Throat complaints and hoarseness; laryngitis.

Sweet tooth: craves sugar, candies, and ice-cream, but all can cause sickness and diarrhea.

Desires salty things, cold drinks, and cold food.

Arnica Arnica montana

COMMON NAMES

LEOPARD'S BANE

Arnica is the pre-eminent remedy for falls and injuries, or for any condition where the person feels as if they were beaten, bruised, injured, or had been run over by a bus, whether this condition is due to illness, lack of sleep, or mental exertion. Sheep seek it out as medicine for their constant injuries in the mountainous areas where it grows.

The Arnica plant has a long history as a healing herb. It grows in mountainous regions of Europe and Siberia.

SYMPTOMS

BETTER for first movement, but worse as movement continues; rest, and lying down with head lower than feet.

WORSE for heat, exposure to hot sun; jarring, lying on injured part, slightest touch, cold, damp, and movement.

REMEDY PROFILE

Despairing and morose; anxious about the future; quarrelsome, opinionated, and obstinate.

Does not want to be approached or touched.

Hopeless and indifferent; in a stupor; forgets words.

Widespread sensations of bruising, soreness, stiffness, and swelling.

Easy bleeding and bruising, externally and internally.

Exhaustion; weariness; sleeplessness; jet lag with bruised, sore feeling.

Shock; trauma.

Sprains, strains, or breaks with pain; inflammation or swelling.

Bed feels hard; sensitive to heat, cold, or touch of any sort.

Use *Arnica* after any injury, accident, fall, operation, or strenuous walk.

Arnica is an invaluable remedy for muscular aches and pains, as well as bruises from falls.

Arsen. alb.

Arsenicum album

People needing Arsen. alb. feel worse for cold drinks and cold foods such as ice cream.

COMMON NAMES

ARSENIC OXIDE

The characteristic symptoms of *Arsenicum* include great restlessness and fear, weakness, and aggravated symptoms at night. Small doses used to be given to horses to make their coats sleek and glossy.

The chief source of the Arsen. alb remedy comes from arsenopyrite, or arsenic ore, which is found in parts of Europe and Canada.

SYMPTOMS

BETTER for company, heat of any kind (except headaches, which are better for fresh air), and changing position.

WORSE for cold, cold food, iced drinks, when alone, and at night (midnight–3.00 am).

REMEDY PROFILE

Pale, thin, anxious perfectionist; has a need for control and order.

Critical and demanding of self and others.

Anxiety about health, germs, possibility of contamination, and time; hates unpunctuality; worries about money, death, and the future.

Fastidious, meticulously clean, and orderly.

Restless: has to move about constantly.

Exhaustion; prostration from minor causes.

Right-sided symptoms.

Extreme sensitivity to cold, but uncomfortable in stuffy rooms.

Burning sensations and pains.

Digestive problems: sickness and diarrhea, indigestion and heartburn, and gastro-enteritis.

Thin, watery (often burning) discharges.

Ulcerative conditions (especially in stomach and bowels) common.

Breathing difficulties common; *Arsen. alb.* is an important asthma remedy.

Heart problems are common, as is high blood pressure.

Dry, scaly skin; eczema.

Thirsty for sips of cold water, but also desires hot drinks; craves oils, fats, and sour foods.

Aurum met.

Aurum metallicum

COMMON NAMES

GOLD

This is an excellent remedy for the person who is over-responsible with a strong sense of duty, and who becomes ill partly as a response to this aspect of their personality.

Gold has been used medicinally for centuries and is still used in medicine and dentistry today. The Aurum met. remedy comes from powdered pure gold.

SYMPTOMS

BETTER for movement, walking in the open air or in sunshine, warm air, summer, and listening to classical music.

WORSE for gloomy days, nightfall, midnight to 2.00 am, 3.00 am and morning, winter, noise, and before menstruation.

REMEDY PROFILE

May have (bloated) red face; congestion; red "drinker's" nose.

Conscientious, responsible, hard-working, meticulous.

Angry; irritable; irascible; easily offended, and cannot bear contradiction.

Critical of self and others; has a strong sense of right and wrong.

Deep depression and self-condemnation.

Dwells on suicide; may plan suicide or jump impulsively from a height.

Many anxieties: about health, about whether he or she has neglected duty or done wrong.

Agoraphobia (fear of open spaces), fear of the dark; fear of heights.

Restless sleep; fixed insomnia; screams in sleep; nightmares.

Pains unbearable; worse at night and when too warm in bed.

Severe bone pain that wanders and disturbs sleep.

Heart and circulation affected: palpitations common, angina pectoris, high blood pressure, hypertension, and stroke.

Great hunger or loss of appetite; thirst for cold drinks.

Chronic indigestion; bilious disorders.

Effects of alcohol and drug abuse; grief, fright, disappointed love, financial loss.

Aurum met. people feel chilly and like to be wrapped up in warm clothes. They feel better for movement and walking in the open air.

People needing Belladonna may suffer from red, hot, itchy skin rashes.

Belladonna Atropa belladonna

COMMON NAMES

DEADLY NIGHTSHADE

The Italian name "beautiful lady" comes from the use of the berries of this poisonous plant as a cosmetic in Venice in the 17th century. Its berries are called "the devil's cherries."

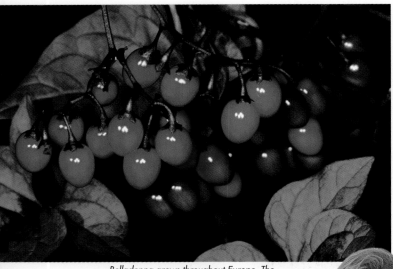

Belladonna grows throughout Europe. The homeopathic remedy is made from the fresh leaves and flowers.

SYMPTOMS

BETTER for pressure, rest, warmth, and light, warm wraps.

WORSE for motion, jarring, touch, pressure, cold, light, noise, 3.00 pm, night, getting head wet, draughts to head, lying on painful side, sun (sunstroke), heat, and lying down.

REMEDY PROFILE

Sudden onset of symptoms; redness; throbbing.

Intense congestions and flushing; throbbing headache; earache; blood vessels and inflamed parts throb and pulse.

Intense emotional state: delirium and mania; sufferer is very restless and agitated, talks very quickly, hallucinates, sees monsters, and lives in his or her own world.

Bad temper, rage, and tantrums.

Skin (mainly head and face) and mucous membranes are bright, shiny red.

Red, hot, dry, itchy, burning skin rashes.

Intense burning and stinging in inflamed parts; very sensitive to touch; everything feels as if about to burst open.

Intense pulsing and throbbing pains, or spasmodic and cramplike; pains begin and end suddenly.

Extreme physical sensitivity; easily affected by jarring, touch, movement, and draughts (especially on head).

Hemorrhages bright-red clotted blood; violent, cramping period pains.

Thirstless usually (but can be thirsty); craves lemons and lemonade.

Complaints are right-sided.

Belladonna people have active, energetic minds. They can experience extremely painful headaches that are made worse by the smallest eye movement.

Bryonia Bryonia alba

COMMON NAMES

WHITE BRYONY OR WILD HOP

The most distinctive characteristic of *Bryonia* is aggravation from motion. Any type of motion makes the symptoms worse, even moving the eyes, in a headache. Its second important characteristic is dryness.

SYMPTOMS

BETTER for firm pressure, lying motionless, cool atmosphere, cold drinks, and compresses.

WORSE for slightest movement, touch, heat (except for local pain, which is better for hot compresses), 3.00 am, 9.00 pm; change from cold to warm or *vice versa*, and exposure to dry cold.

REMEDY PROFILE

Extremely irritable; touchy; morose.

Wants to be at work; does not want to talk or be interfered with in any way.

Anxious about money, security, and business.

Discontented, yet does not know what he or she wants; children ask for things and then reject what is offered.

Dryness of mucous membranes; constipation: large, hard, dry, crumbly stools.

Dry, racking, irritating, painful cough (worse for movement and warm rooms); thirsty for long drinks of cold water; colds go to chest.

Dryness of fluids lubricating joints; stitches; tearing pains with swelling: better for rest and pressure and tight bandaging, and worse for movement.

Dryness in digestive system; bitter taste; tongue coated white/yellow; stomach fluids dry up and food lies like a stone; nausea and vomiting.

Symptoms right-sided.

Headache with all illnesses; vertigo.

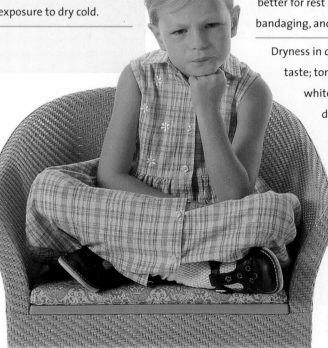

Children needing Bryonia can be difficult to please: they may ask for things yet reject them when they are offered. Usually they do not want to be lifted or carried.

Calc. carb. Calcarea carbonica

COMMON NAMES

CALCIUM CARBONATE

People who need this remedy are physically and mentally weak, easily tired, and tend to sweat from the slightest exertion. It is commonly used for people who are plump and fair-skinned, who have poor muscle tone and are prone to swollen lymphs.

The Calc. carb. remedy is prepared from calcium carbonate, which comes from the shell of the European oyster.

SYMPTOMS

BETTER for dry weather and being constipated.

WORSE for cold of all kinds, intellectual or physical effort, and the full moon.

People needing the Calc. carb. remedy may have a craving for milk or may detest it. When they drink it, it will have a tendency to upset the digestion.

REMEDY PROFILE

Emotionally vulnerable; full of fears and anxieties.

Lack of confidence; timidity; can be extremely self-conscious.

Extremely anxious and fearful: many phobias and fears about failing, health, the dark, and insanity.

Closed and reserved; hides fears and anxiety.

Methodical, practical, orderly, hard worker.

Obstinate and cannot be hurried.

Weakness; easily fatigued.

Flabby tissues and a tendency to put on weight (but can be thin).

Poor circulation; feels chilly and is sensitive to cold and damp.

Sweats easily; cold sweat and clammy handshake; children (and sometimes adults) sweat profusely around head and scalp.

Slow development as child, with tendency to catch colds, get sore throats, tonsillitis, and illnesses involving the glands.

In later life, prone to develop new growths (polyps and bony growths).

Craves indigestible foods such as coal, chalk, and raw potatoes; also craves eggs, sweet things, and ice-cream; desires (or detests) milk.

Digestion worse for milk; often hungry; thirst may be marked.

Causticum is a potassium compound that is prepared by distilling burned lime, water, and potassium bisulphate.

Causticum

Causticum hahnemanni

COMMON NAMES

POTASSIUM HYDRATE

For a person in a melancholy and anxious state, bleak in mood and tearful. It is one of only three remedies whose symptoms are better for wet weather. The others are *Nux vomica* and *Hepar sulf*. People who need *Causticum* can often tell when rain is on the way by the increase in their aches and pains, which improve when the weather breaks.

SYMPTOMS

BETTER for cold drinks, damp wet weather, washing, and warmth of bed.

WORSE for dry, cold, or raw air, winds, draughts, extremes of temperature, fats, 3.00–4.00 am, evening, change of weather, darkness, burns, fright, and grief.

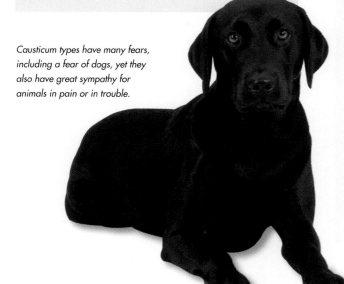

Causticum types have many fears, including a fear of dogs, yet they also have great sympathy for animals in pain or in trouble.

REMEDY PROFILE

Paralysis; paralysing anxiety and fear (worse at twilight and night); lack of self-confidence; timidity.

Paralysis of confidence and will; extremely cautious.

Suicidal from thinking about anxiety and fears.

Foreboding; apprehension; jumps at least noise.

Fears on waking; fears of dogs, evil, ghosts, and the future; children do not want to go to bed alone.

Anxiety for others; deeply concerned about injustice, especially children; intense sympathy with people, animals in pain or trouble.

Caustic and sarcastic; censorious and critical.

Quarrelsome, peevish, and incensed at trifles.

Pessimism, depression, and anxiety; sudden tears and floods of emotion; long-lasting grief.

Worn-out constitution; stiff joints; chronic rheumatic problems causing contraction of tendons; deformities around joints.

Restlessness of legs at night.

Paralysis of single parts of body (Parkinson's, Bell's Palsy); small paralyses of throat with difficulty swallowing; paralysis of the eyelid, causing drooping.

Headaches with facial neuralgia.

Cystitis, sensitive to cold, incontinence, worse for coughing and sneezing.

Effects of burns and scalds.

Chamomilla
Matricaria recutita

COMMON NAMES

GERMAN CAMOMILE

P eople who need *Chamomilla* are probably the most irritable and irascible in existence. Nothing pleases them. It is a very good choice for a toddler who has frequent temper tantrums.

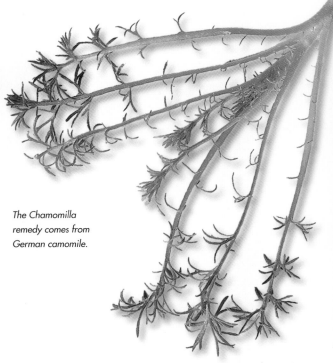

The Chamomilla remedy comes from German camomile.

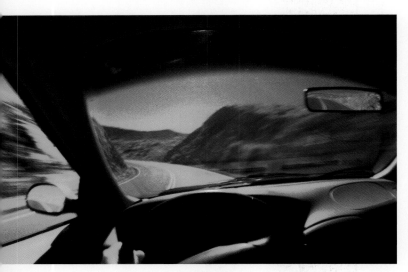

Chamomilla people feel better for traveling in cars.

SYMPTOMS

BETTER for being carried, traveling in car, heat (except toothache), and warm, humid weather.

WORSE for draughts, wind, wet, anger, 9.00 pm to midnight, coffee, narcotics, and also before and during periods.

REMEDY PROFILE

Sensitivity to pain; pain unbearable.

Angry; complaints resulting from anger; restlessness; temper tantrums.

This is the most irritable and irascible of remedy pictures; nothing is right.

Easily offended; refuses to reply when spoken to.

Restless from pain and anger.

Little appetite.

Marked thirst for cold water; desire for acid drinks.

Attacks of severe vomiting with retching; bilious from anger.

Slimy, green diarrhea.

Sleep disturbed and restless; nightmares; hot in bed.

Sweats easily and feels better for sweating.

Sensitive to wind, chill from damp, cold air and cold.

Teething problems.

China

China officinalis/cinchona succinibra

The China remedy is made from the Peruvian bark tree, and was the first substance that Hahnemann tested on himself.

COMMON NAMES

CINCHONA, PERUVIAN BARK

A person who needs *China* will be exhausted, irritable, touchy, or apathetic when ill. The illness may have been brought on by prolonged mental strain or conditions involving loss of body fluids: diarrhea, sickness, and heavy blood loss are some more severe examples.

SYMPTOMS

BETTER for firm pressure, warmth, and sleep.

WORSE for slightest touch, draughts, cold air, movement, night (especially midnight), fall, and eating fruit or acid things.

REMEDY PROFILE

Pale; dark circles around eyes.

Exhausted; edgy and irritable.

Apathetic; disinclined to make intellectual effort.

Dislikes company or activity.

Timid and anxious, especially at night.

Fears dogs and crawling insects.

Sensitive to noise and external impressions.

Chilly; sensitive to colds and draughts; worse for cold weather and fresh air.

Flushes of heat and bouts of shivering.

Bloating, gas, and distension; painless, watery diarrhea; green, watery, corroding stools, with colic.

Hungry, but quickly feels full.

Craves condiments, stimulants, and alcohol.

Averse to butter and fatty foods; intolerant of sour things, fish, fruit, wine, and milk.

Diarrhea after consuming milk and fruit (especially infants).

Hemorrhages; frequent nosebleeds; periods heavy with dark, clotted blood.

Sleepy during day, but cannot sleep at night; restless, especially early at night; vivid, distressing dreams disturb sleep.

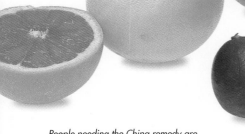

People needing the China remedy are intolerant of sour and acid foods and feel worse for eating citrus fruit.

Gelsemium

Gelsemium sempervirens

COMMON NAMES

YELLOW JASMINE, WILD WOODBINE

Yellow jasmine is the source of the homeopathic remedy Gelsemium. The chopped root of the plant is soaked in alcohol to make a tincture.

Drowsiness and mental and physical weakness are the prominent symptoms of the person needing *Gelsemium*. Its plant source, the jasmine, cannot stand up without being supported on canes or trellises—so the *Gelsemium* person may need to lean on others for help.

SYMPTOMS

BETTER for movement, sweating, and urination.

WORSE for heat, hot weather, bad news, anticipation, excitement, and physical exertion.

REMEDY PROFILE

Major remedy for influenza.

Severe anticipatory anxiety about many things, including death, crowds, open spaces, falling, exams, and public appearances; trembles; becomes paralysed, heavy, and sluggish.

Sluggish depression; wants to be alone, yet hates isolation.

Nervous exhaustion; trembling; weakness; paralysed sensation in limbs; feels completely drained.

Weariness and heaviness; needs to lie down; wilts and collapses.

Gradual onset of feverish states; chills and flushed face; internal chills, as if cold water running down back; dazed; delirious.

Congestive headaches with pain at the back and bottom of head.

Dullness and blurring of vision, sometimes double vision, especially with headaches.

Nervous diarrhea.

Thirstless.

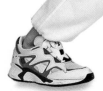
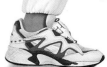

Gelsemium people feel worse for physical exertion and their fears and phobias may prevent them from leading an active life.

Hepar sulf.

Hepar sulfuris calcareum

The Hepar sulf. remedy is also known as calcium sulfide. It is prepared from a mixture of calcium carbonate from oyster shells and powdered sulfur.

COMMON NAMES

CALCIUM SULFIDE

Hepar sulf's outstanding characteristic is its capacity to respond to and help extreme sensitivity of every sort, to touch, cold, emotion, and pain. All troubles and physical symptoms are better for wet weather.

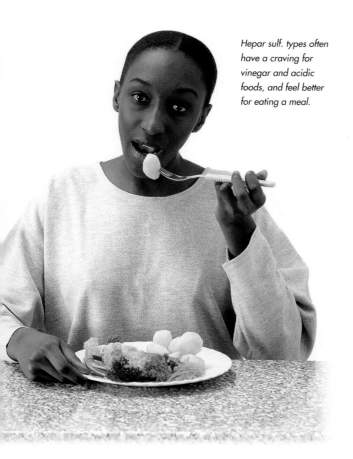

Hepar sulf. types often have a craving for vinegar and acidic foods, and feel better for eating a meal.

REMEDY PROFILE

Emotionally oversensitive; touchy, irritable, impatient, quarrelsome, angry, and abusive.

Hasty and impulsive; ready to burst out.

Impulses to commit suicide.

Physically oversensitive: to touch, surroundings, pain, cold, and the least draught.

Infected parts extremely tender to touch: cannot even bear bedclothes.

Slightest pressure causes sharp pain, as if a splinter.

Everything festers and suppurates (gathers or discharges pus); feels sore, as if a boil.

Catarrhal states prominent; catarrhal colds.

Splintering pains in throat or sensation as of a lodged fishbone.

Facial neuralgia; often right-sided after exposure to cold wind.

Thick, cheesy, yellow discharges.

Sour, offensive sweats.

SYMPTOMS

BETTER for eating a meal, staying warm, and wrapping up the head.

WORSE for cold, especially dry cold.

Ignatia

Ignatia amara/strychnos ignatii

COMMON NAMES
ST IGNATIUS' BEAN

Ignatia is known as the funeral remedy because of the similarity of its symptom picture to expressions of grief and its helpfulness to people in this state. It is derived from the St Ignatius Bean, the bitter and poisonous seed of a pear-shaped fruit native to the Philippines. Like *Nux vomica*, it is one of the main sources of strychnine. The two remedies have a lot of characteristics in common.

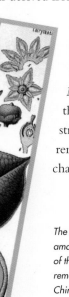

The seeds of the Ignatia amara tree are the source of this homeopathic remedy. They grow in China and the East Indies.

SYMPTOMS

BETTER socializing, having a good time, and exposure to heat.

WORSE for mornings (especially 11.00 am), unpleasant emotions, consolation, strong smells, grief, shock, fear, and disappointments in love.

REMEDY PROFILE

Reserved, but suddenly bursts out with emotions.

Sensitive; moody; emotional; irritable and angry.

Great upset; "hysterical" reactions; laughs and cries in turn; easily melancholy; tearful; disposed to mull over problems.

Hypersensitive to bad news.

Dread, fear, and anxiety are common.

Fear of being trapped or constricted.

Any physical symptoms that come on through high emotion or upset: headache, migraine, nausea, fainting, cough, and colic.

Spasmodic conditions such as twitching and jerking of muscles; spastic colon; hiccoughs; spasmodic cough.

Fleeting, erratic pains.

Temporary paralysis or numbness without apparent cause.

Oversensitive to smells, pain, and noise.

Frequent deep sighing or yawning.

Sensation of lump in the throat.

Paradoxical symptoms: indigestion that improves on eating; pain in throat, which is worse for liquids but not for solid foods; hunger not relieved by eating; and pain better for pressure.

Use for effects of grief, separation, and shock.

Ipecacuanha (Ipecac)
Cephaelis ipecacuanha

COMMON NAMES

IPECACUANHA

Ipecac is made from the roots of a Brazilian creeping plant brought to Europe by the Portuguese in the late seventeenth century. The Portuguese name means "sick–making plant." It was used as a remedy for hemorrages and nausea for centuries, and is still found in cough medicines.

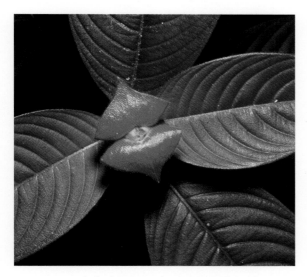

Cephaelis ipecacuanha is a perennial shrub that grows in rain forests. The dried root is used to make the Ipecac. remedy.

SYMPTOMS

BETTER for firm pressure, open air, and rest.

WORSE for cold weather, excessive heat, damp weather, veal, pork, and ices.

REMEDY PROFILE

Hard to please; peevish, irritable, impatient, and scornful.

Sporadic patches of exhaustion and prostration.

Acute nausea; most complaints accompanied by nausea.

Acute attacks of difficult breathing.

Acute bleeding accompanies many complaints.

Chilly; thirstless.

Cough, colds, and bronchitis.

Headaches at the back of the head , accompanied by nausea; neuralgic pains in eye.

Strong desire for candies, which can cause the characteristic green, slimy diarrhea.

Periods are too early and too frequent; bright-red clotted blood with faintness; bleeding between periods: bright-red, gushing, and worse for movement.

Extreme nausea in pregnancy, probably with excessive salivation.

Profuse bleeding during and after labor.

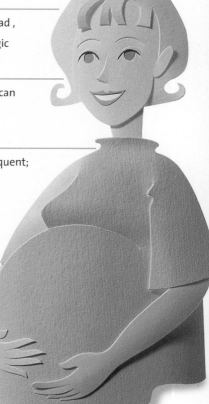

Kali carb.

Kali carbonicum

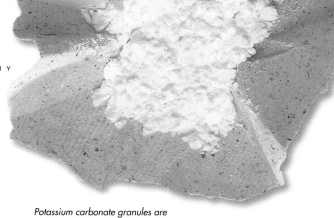

Potassium carbonate granules are triturated or dissolved in purified water in order to produce the remedy Kali carb.

POTASSIUM CARBONATE

This is the only remedy with puffiness and swelling of the upper eyelids. Also extremely characteristic are exhausation, low back pain, fear felt in the stomach, extreme sensitivity to light touch and the effects of missing a meal.

SYMPTOMS

BETTER for warm, open air and warmth of any kind.

WORSE for cold, chill, damp, pressure, fast movement, any exertion (especially sexual), not eating, getting too hot, and at 2.00–5.00am.

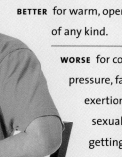

Kali carb. people are easily exhausted and feel worse for mental or physical exertion. They have weak muscles and ligaments, especially in the lower back.

REMEDY PROFILE

Timid and apprehensive; easily frightened, especially of dogs and the dark.

Fear of being alone; feels anxious and worries about everything, including poverty, health, death, and the future.

Nervy and irritable; easily startled.

Easily aggravated by noise and disorder.

Understates emotions and overexplains.

Falls asleep, especially after eating and over food.

Stitching pains can occur anywhere: worse for rest or motion, or lying on affected side.

Digestive problems: flatulence, acid risings, distension, sour belching, constipation, and feelings of emptiness.

Craves candies, sugar, and starchy foods.

Feels worse for missing a meal; anxious when hungry.

Periods profuse and exhausting; cycle may be long.

Patient extremely sensitive to cold, damp, draughts, and cold air.

Kidneys weak; general waterlogged state; swelling of upper eyelids.

Sweaty from slightest exertion.

Predominantly right-sided symptoms.

Cannot sleep or wakes between 2.00 and 5.00 am; disturbing dreams.

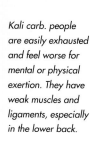

Lachesis Trigonocephalus lachesis/lachesis muta

Lachesis people are passionate, excitable, and extrovert, but can suffer from mood swings.

COMMON NAMES

BUSHMASTER OR SURUKUKU

Lachesis is left-sided, the eyes flicker like a snake's, the person is always worse after sleep, is sensitive to the slightest pressure (mental or physical), and everything is better for flow and expression. The mental state is almost "volcanic."

SYMPTOMS

BETTER for discharge of any kind, including feelings, ideas, and flow of body fluids; moderate temperatures and fresh air.

WORSE for suppression, constriction, restriction, delayed or suppressed periods, heat generally, being touched, after sleep, and during the spring.

The Lachesis remedy comes from the venom of the South American bushmaster snake.

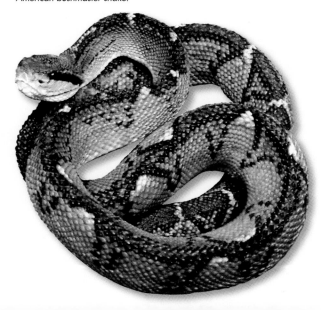

REMEDY PROFILE

Passionate, intense, excitable nature; extrovert; talkative; animated.

Mood swings: alternates between excitement and depression.

Restless depression, with anxiety.

Deeply affected by loss and bereavement.

Jealousy; spitefulness; high sex drive.

Psychic tendencies; disturbing dreams.

Suspicious: feels plotted against.

Worse after sleep and on waking.

Left-sided symptoms, or start on left and move to right.

Hypersensitive to light, noise, touch, and heat.

Cannot bear constriction round throat or abdomen.

Warm-blooded; worse for heat and stuffy rooms.

Circulation affected: bluish-purple color in veins and skin.

All symptoms worse before periods, but better when flow is established.

Menopause a crucial period: great difficulties.

Alcoholic tendencies.

Lycopodium
Lycopodium clavatum

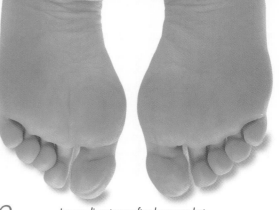

Lycopodium types often have one hot foot and one cold foot. They hate the cold, but are wearied by heat.

The person in need of *Lycopodium* always seems confident and domineering, but inside is anxious and insecure, fearful of being "found out." He or she is anxious in social situations, but at the same time fears being alone.

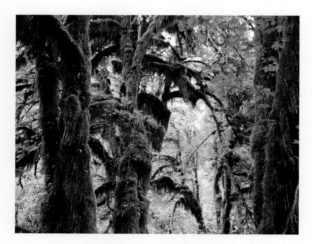

The Lycopodium remedy comes from club moss, which grows in forests. Homeopaths use pollen dust extracted from the spikes.

SYMPTOMS

BETTER for cool, open air, being busy, hot foods and drinks, warmth, and loose clothes.

WORSE for being contradicted, cold foods or drinks, 4.00–8.00 pm, on waking, hot stuffy atmospheres, emotional stress, worry, and old age.

REMEDY PROFILE

Mixture of cowardice and arrogance, timidity and authority; pleasant manner, but angry, blustering, and tyrannical at home.

Deeply furrowed brow; strong feeling of anxious anticipation, but performs well.

Fearful and panicky: fears crowds, closed places, going outside, darkness, illness, death, being found out, undertaking anything and not reaching destination.

Outbursts of temper; dwells on resentments.

Depressed; detached; seemingly haughty.

Fear of commitment and rejection.

Likes to be alone with someone in the next room.

Sentimental, and weeps when thanked.

Psychosexual problems in men.

Right-sided symptoms, extending to left.

Many digestive symptoms: hungry, but full after a few mouthfuls; bloated and flatulent soon after eating; no relief from wind or burping.

Craves sugar, sweet things, and hot foods and drinks; intolerant of cabbage, beans, onions, oysters, pastry.

Cannot stand clothes tight around waist.

Tendency to colds, bronchitis, and pneumonia.

General physical awkwardness and weakness, with poor muscle tone.

Merc. Sol.

Mercurius solubilis hahnemanni

BELOW *The Merc. sol. remedy comes from cinnabar, an ore of mercury, which is found in the US, Europe, and China.*

COMMON NAMES

MERCURY

Mercurcius is quicksilver, the only metal that is liquid at room temperature. It trembles when it liquifies, and the person who needs it also trembles or shakes a great deal, being influenced by almost all environments.

SYMPTOMS

BETTER for moderate temperatures.

WORSE for extremes of temperature, changes of temperature, sweating, right side, and night.

Merc. sol. people have an aversion to meat, fat, and butter, and suffer from stomach upsets after eating candies.

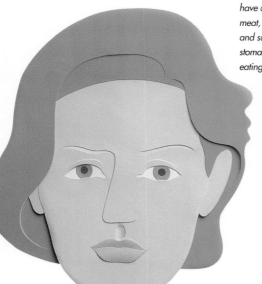

REMEDY PROFILE

Anxiety, fear, and apprehension.

Hasty and hurried; restless and impulsive.

Nervous children; inclined to stutter.

Depression and confusion; poor comprehension; bad memory.

Time passes slowly; weary; disillusioned.

Glands: especially salivary glands and glands of throat and neck.

Wounds quickly gather and discharge pus, with burning and stinging; yellow or yellowish-green pus.

Repeated ear infections with offensive pus discharges.

Abscesses in the glands and the roots of the teeth.

Ulceration, especially of mucous membranes, as in mouth ulcers, stomach ulcers, and colitis.

Foul-smelling breath, and spongy, yellow-white gums, which tend to ulcerate; general redness and ulceration of mouth and throat.

Tongue has thick, yellow coating, is swollen, and shows marks of teeth on its sides.

Metallic or sweet or salty taste; insatiable hunger and sense of dryness with intense thirst, especially for milk and beer.

Increased saliva; perspiration profuse and smelly.

Natrum mur.

Natrum muriaticum

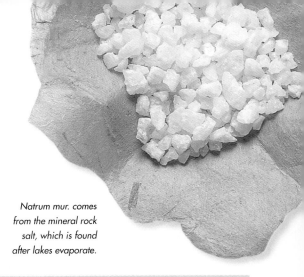

Natrum mur. comes from the mineral rock salt, which is found after lakes evaporate.

COMMON NAMES

SODIUM CHLORIDE, SEA SALT

Nat mur is a remedy for when the body fluid balance of the body is disturbed. The character needing this remedy is reserved, introverted, difficult to get to know, aggravated by consolation; tends to live in the past and likes to reminisce over old times and memories.

SYMPTOMS

BETTER for open air, not eating (despite good appetite), and being at the seaside.

WORSE for consolation, 10.00 am, intellectual work, direct heat, sun, full moon, extremes of temperature, stress, overexcitement, and quinine.

REMEDY PROFILE

Thin; pale-skinned; the lower lip is often cracked vertically in the center.

Reserved and self-contained; wary of emotional involvement; fears being hurt emotionally; falls in love with unavailable people.

Fears betrayal and rejection.

Hangs on to past disappointments, hurts, and resentments; bears grudges.

Averse to sympathy and consolation; cries alone.

Fears: robbers, darkness, heights, closed spaces, losing control, and being laughed at.

Depression; loathing of life, but bears with it.

Feels guilt and remorse easily.

Suppresses anger.

Emotional breakdown from prolonged stress.

Exhaustion after small effort.

Prone to herpes.

Disturbed fluid balance and retains water in several different forms; edema (swelling); premenstrual syndrome; severe constipation; mucus formation; greasy skin and hair; headaches.

Sensitive to cold.

Good appetite; intense thirst for water or tea.

Craves/hates salt and salty foods, and bread.

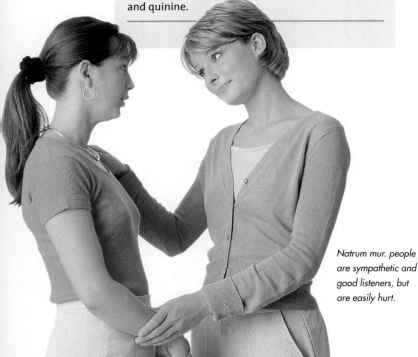

Natrum mur. people are sympathetic and good listeners, but are easily hurt.

Nux vomica

Strychnos nux vomica

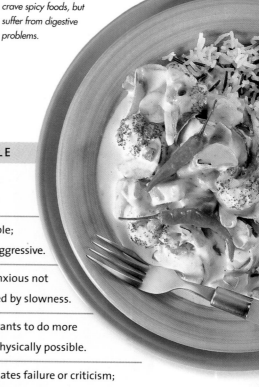

Nux vomica people crave spicy foods, but suffer from digestive problems.

COMMON NAMES

POISON NUT, VOMITING NUT

Nux vomica is made from the seed of the poisonous nut *Strychnos nux vomica*, from which strychnine comes. It is a good cleanser of the system after the person has been taking a lot of medicines. It is stronger than *Ignatia*.

SYMPTOMS

BETTER for sleep, heat, night, and wet weather.

WORSE for cold and dry weather, wind, stimulants, after meals, morning, on waking, and between 3.00 and 4.00 am.

Nux vomica is prepared from the seeds of the poison nut tree.

REMEDY PROFILE

Lively and responsive; active and engaged.

Tense; impatient; irritable; competitive; excitable; aggressive.

Impatient; in a hurry; anxious not to waste time; frustrated by slowness.

Perfectionist; orderly; wants to do more than emotionally and physically possible.

Pride easily wounded; hates failure or criticism; emotionally sensitive; touchy; quick to take offense.

Anxiety about work, the future, health, and security.

Suicidal thoughts; fear of knives and impulse to kill with them; sudden impulses to violence.

Craves alcohol, spicy foods, fats, condiments, coffee.

Digestive problems tending to constipation (wants to pass stools but cannot) and piles; biliousness; sensitive to cold, but dislikes stuffy atmospheres.

Hates wind; edgy before thunderstorms.

Nervous twitches; spasmodic movements, sneezing.

Oversensitive nervous system: reacts sharply and quickly to cold, bright light, slightest noise, smells, and pollens. Many allergic reactions.

Unbearable shooting, tearing, stitching pains.

Excess of all kinds of appetites; overuses stimulants, alcohol, and tranquilizers. Useful in addictions.

Phosphorus people are often artistic, sensitive, and intuitive.

Phos. Phosphorus

COMMON NAMES

WHITE PHOSPHORUS

Phosphorus, in its natural form, must be kept under water, or it will burst into flames. The person needing it is sensitive to all impressions, quickly aroused, easily inflamed with buring sensations.

Phos. derives from the mineral white phosphorus— a highly unstable material.

SYMPTOMS

BETTER for heat, sleep, and eating.

WORSE for cold, storms, lightning, lying on the left side, twilight, walking quickly, and loss of vital fluids.

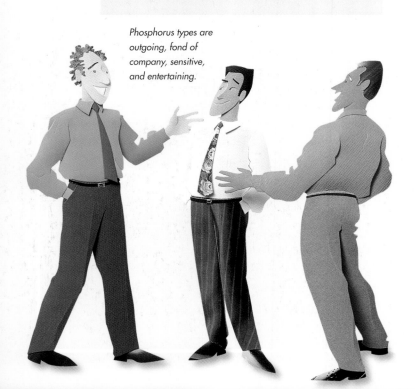

Phosphorus types are outgoing, fond of company, sensitive, and entertaining.

REMEDY PROFILE

Tall and slender; general lack of physical energy.

Rapid growth when young, but tendency to weakness.

Needs close contact physically and emotionally.

Needs attention and reassurance.

Lives in the moment; short attention span.

Impressionable; oversensitive to emotional atmospheres, light, noise, and smells.

A psychic sponge: takes ghosts and spirits for granted.

Sympathetic: identifies with thoughts and feelings of others, but loses sense of separate identity.

Intuitive thinker; artistic and dramatic.

Very sensual, but worse for excessive sexual activity.

Intense imagination; anxious dreams; sleepwalks.

Alternation between excitement and depression, and between high energy and apathetic collapse.

Depression, despondency, and suicidal despair.

Easily startled; full of fears: of the future; being alone, especially at night; disease and death; thunder, lightning; illness, and impending misfortune.

Bleeding that begins easily: nosebleeds, menstrual and rectal bleeding; blood from lungs, ulcers, or gums.

Burning sensations, especially in palms.

Craving for salt, salty foods, and cold foods and drinks (but nauseous when they become warm in stomach).

Desire to eat at 3.00 am; aversion to sweet foods, meat, tea, boiled milk, salted fish, and oysters.

Pulsatilla Pulsatilla nigricans/ anemone pratensis

The perennial Pulsatilla nigricans plant, or wind flower, is the source of the homeopathic remedy Pulsatilla.

COMMON NAMES

WIND FLOWER, MEADOW ANEMONE

Pulsatilla is very often useful for children's moods or when adults fall into states more usual with children—sulking or moaning, for example. Its source, the windflower, grows in dry places, in groups, is easily shaken by the wind, and often droops its head. Changeability is the keynote: of both the moods of the patient and the symptoms.

SYMPTOMS

BETTER for gentle motion, fresh air, pregnancy, sympathy, consolation, and company.

WORSE for being alone, bereavement, change, unfamiliar surroundings, evening, twilight, morning, heat, stuffy rooms, rich and fatty foods, sudden chill, and getting wet.

Pulsatilla types are charming, pleasant, mild-natured, emotional, and affectionate. They are also timid and dislike confrontations or giving offense.

REMEDY PROFILE

Dependent nature: wants support, reassurance, and company; cries easily and feels better for crying.

Touchy, easily hurt; discontented, indecisive, demanding, needy; jealous and distrustful.

Depression; sadness; loneliness; changeable.

Fears being alone, especially in the evening, and being abandoned, unloved, and helpless; also fears the dark, ghosts, crowds, open spaces, illness, domestic troubles, and going insane.

Flushes easily; one part of body hot, another cold.

Pains variable: rheumatic pains wander from one part of body to another. Discharges are bland, creamy yellow or greenish-yellow.

Catarrhal conditions; long-lasting head colds, resulting in deafness; earaches; rhinitis.

Sticky or stuck eyes in the morning; conjunctivitis; styes.

Menstrual periods delayed, scanty, and painful; periods easily stop: caused by anorexia, going abroad, and upsets.

Varicose veins, chilblains, piles, constipation, and cold extremities.

Thirstless; craves butter, pastries, creamy foods, yet upset by them.

Nausea, vomiting, and heartburn.

Rhus tox.

Rhus toxicodendron/r. radicans

COMMON NAMES

POISON IVY OR POISON OAK

The most distinctive characteristic of the *Rhus tox.* picture is that symptoms are relieved by gradual movement, especially the arthritic and rheumatic pain and restless anxiety characteristic of the person needing the remedy.

SYMPTOMS

BETTER for slow, continued movement, warm and dry weather, clothes, hot drinks, and hot applications.

WORSE for getting wet, change of weather to cold/damp, during fall, getting chilled, cold drinks and food; damp, draughts, first movement, rest, sitting, lying down, and evening, especially at around 7.00 pm.

REMEDY PROFILE

Anxiety and mental restlessness; seems to worry about everything.

Worries about future, family, business.

Nervous and irritable; sadness.

Thoughts of suicide and weary of life.

Physical restlessness.

Painful stiffness of muscles and joints; shooting, tearing pains.

Pains worse for first movement, but better for slow, continued motion.

Tongue has triangular red tip in illness.

Blister-like eruptions appear on skin; herpes.

Skin red and itchy, burning, and swollen, especially at night or if hot.

Unquenchable thirst for cold drinks.

Desire for candie, cold milk, and cold drinks; dislikes meat and bread.

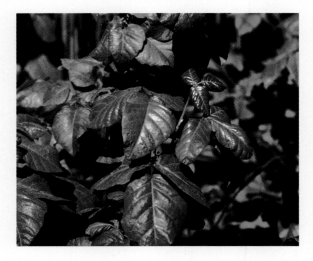

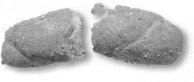
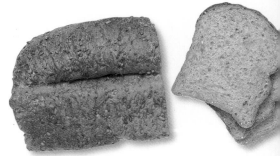

The Rhus tox. remedy comes from the fresh leaves of poison ivy, which grows in the US and Canada.

Sepia

Sepia officinalis

COMMON NAMES

CUTTLEFISH, SQUID INK

The squid moves very quickly, jetting through the water at high speed; it also pours out a brown liquid to protect itself, spreading a protective gloom through the surrounding water. People who need *Sepia* have a brown, depressive mood; they also look brown with sallow skin and brown patches.

Sepia people crave chocolate, and bitter, acidic, and spicy foods, but have a strong dislike of fats and milk.

SYMPTOMS

BETTER for strenuous exercise, dancing, fast walking, and occupation.

WORSE for stuffy rooms, cold air, evening, night, rest, standing or kneeling for long periods, atmosphere before a storm, sexual intercourse, and clothes too tight round neck and abdomen.

REMEDY PROFILE

Energetic, active, busy, and purposeful, or burned out, collapsed, and depleted.

Feels trapped and wants to escape; profound depression; suicidal, dragged down.

Sags and droops mentally and physically; stagnation; cannot be bothered: feels worn out.

Fears of death, poverty, starvation, humiliation, ghosts, and thunderstorms.

Strongly indicated at times of hormonal change: menses, pregnancy, menopause, after abortion, and post-natal depression.

Weepy and irritable; impatient; silent and moody.

Indifferent to everyone and everything, including family, loved ones, and sex.

General chilliness, with poor circulation.

General pelvic weakness and lack of tone in veins and muscles, as if insides would fall out; prolapse; varicose veins; piles.

Menopausal problems: hot flushes, dryness.

Tendency to constipation; backache; weariness.

Sensation of lump or ball in various parts of body.

Left-sided symptoms.

Likes bitter, tart foods, including vinegar and pickles, and acidic, spicy, or highly seasoned foods; strong aversion to fats and milk; craves chocolate.

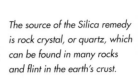

The source of the Silica remedy is rock crystal, or quartz, which can be found in many rocks and flint in the earth's crust.

Silica Silicea terra

COMMON NAMES

SILICON DIOXIDE, QUARTZ, FLINT, SAND

A grain of quartz sand is very hard and gritty; it takes a long process to bring it to its present inflexible form. The person needing *Silica* embodies these qualities of hardness, granularity, rigidity, and continuity on both their mental and physical planes.

SYMPTOMS

BETTER for heat, warm clothing, summer, and lying down.

WORSE for cold, draughts, before and during thunderstorms, exertion, and vaccinations.

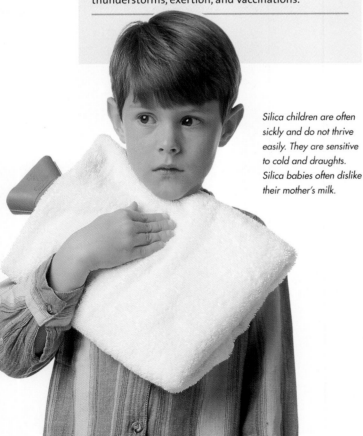

Silica children are often sickly and do not thrive easily. They are sensitive to cold and draughts. Silica babies often dislike their mother's milk.

REMEDY PROFILE

Low physical and mental energy, born tired; lacks stamina; easily fatigued and affected by stress.

Cautious, timid, diffident, unassertive; low self-confidence; intolerant of criticism or contradiction.

Intellectual burnout; loses concentration.

Fears: not being able to carry on, being away from home, needles, knives, sharp-pointed objects, driving, and being robbed.

Easily discouraged and indecisive; worries over trifles.

Usually yields to others, but strong-willed, determined, and obstinate where fact or principle is important.

Fastidious; conscientious; doggedly persevering, and works hard, yet dreads responsibility and is reluctant to undertake anything for fear of failure.

Anxious anticipation, long in advance of event.

Sleeplessness, especially away from home.

Terrifying dreams; tendency to sleepwalking.

Easily startled; jumps if touched; irritated by trifles.

Sensitivity to colds and draughts.

Repeated colds, possibly developing into bronchitis.

Drenching head sweats; smelly, sweaty feet.

Slightest wound gathers and discharges pus; boils; abscesses; sensation of splinters or needles in skin.

Great thirst, but poor appetite; frequently does not assimilate nutrients from food; may become thin.

Craves cold food; dislikes hot food and meat.

Staphysagria

Delphinium staphysagria

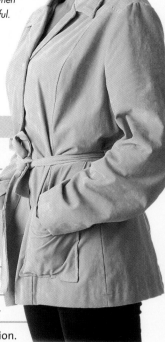

Staphysagria people are very likeable and agreeable, but they hide their feelings when hurt and may feel resentful.

COMMON NAMES

STAVESACRE, LARKSPUR

People who need *Staphysagria* are very sensitive, physically, and emotionally. If they have been hurt badly, they tend to hold onto the pain, but behave in a mild, pleasant way until it gets too much, when they may burst out in an explosion of temper. It is an important remedy for the effects, acute and long-term, of bullying or abuse.

The seeds from the Delphinium staphysagria plant are dried, ground, and soaked in alcohol to produce this remedy.

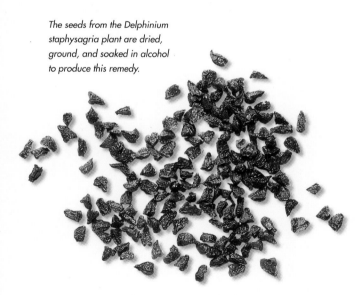

SYMPTOMS

BETTER for rest, eating, and warmth.

WORSE for exertion, sexual excess, suppressed anger, touch, tobacco, and early morning.

REMEDY PROFILE

Very agreeable personality.

Occasional glimpse of resentment or hurt and indignation.

Hides feelings when hurt and pretends nothing has happened.

Self-righteous; sensitive to hurt; touchy.

Reserved displeasure; silent indignation.

Deep feelings of worthlessness/depression.

Fears: not being good enough, failure, and being unlovable or worthless, abandoned, or hurt.

Displaced or suppressed anger; resentment; loss of voice when angry; suicidal depression.

Sexual fantasies, also decreased interest in sex.

Exhaustion; trembling from suppressed emotions.

Sighing, especially when swallowing.

Weeping eczema; coughs; headaches; cystitis; stomach ache; toothache; wounds painful and heal slowly.

Sensitive, bleeding gums; teeth black from decay.

Prey to mosquitoes and other biting insects.

Increased or decreased menstruation; bleeding stops after upset; postmenopausal bleeding.

Great hunger, even after eating; craves bread, milk, and tobacco; generally thirstless.

Sulfur Sulfur

The source of the Sulfur remedy is a fine yellow powder, which is extracted from the mineral sulfur.

COMMON NAMES

BRIMSTONE, BURNING STONE

People who need *Sulfur* can be enthusiastic, sociable, open-hearted extroverts or introverted academic types, who are full of energy and ideas for many projects, which they never complete because something else comes along. They are warm-blooded and very sensitive to heat.

SYMPTOMS

BETTER for motion and fresh air; naps.

WORSE for being still (especially when standing), heat in bed, severe cold, washing, 11.00 am, waking, during spring.

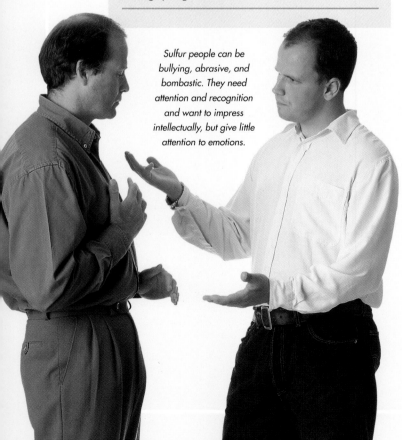

Sulfur people can be bullying, abrasive, and bombastic. They need attention and recognition and want to impress intellectually, but give little attention to emotions.

REMEDY PROFILE

Eccentric, red-faced, untidy person; red rims to orifices, itchy skin.

Can be easy-going, hospitable, entertaining, or can be a self-centered bore, constantly talking, theorizing, full of ideas and plans that go nowhere.

Restless and driven, or depressed, apathetic, lazy, dissatisfied, can drop out, go on the road.

Quarrelsome, critical, irritable over trifles, uncooperative, argues. Morose, grumpy.

Ideas and thoughts prevent sleep, or wakes 3.00–5.00 am; sleep unrefreshing, drowsy during day.

Anxiety about future, health, disease, and religion.

Warm-blooded and red-faced; uncomfortable in heated rooms or spaces, especially during menopause.

Craving for fresh air; dislike of extreme cold.

Burning sensations and pains, especially burning in soles of feet at night, and burning on top of head.

Dry, rough, itchy skin with tendency to eruptions, sores, and pus spots; scratches until it bleeds.

Frequent hunger, especially around 11.00 am; sinking feeling from hunger.

Craves or dislikes fat, salt, candie, spicy foods, and pickles; marked thirst, especially for water and alcohol.

Digestive discomfort: diarrhea that drives the person from bed in early morning; piles.

Offensive discharges, body odor.

Thuja types cannot digest onions or fat, and rarely eat breakfast.

Thuja Thuja occidentalis

COMMON NAMES

TREE OF LIFE, ARBOR VITAE, WHITE CEDAR

The *Thuja* tree grows in Northern Europe and the northern states of America. Nowadays, it provides wood for poles and fences these days. This gives us a clue to the *Thuja* personality, which is one of the most fixed and rigid in the *Materia Medica*.

SYMPTOMS

BETTER for cool air and perspiration.

WORSE for exposure to damp, cold, heat in bed, 3.00 am, 3.00 pm, onions, tea, menstruation, full moon, and vaccinations.

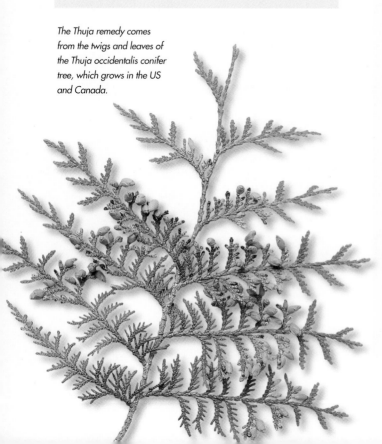

The Thuja remedy comes from the twigs and leaves of the Thuja occidentalis conifer tree, which grows in the US and Canada.

REMEDY PROFILE

Pale; fleshy; greasy complexion; retains water.

Fixed and rigid personality: obsessional; fixed ideas.

Striking caution and reserve; closed; mistrustful; wary.

Little self-confidence; fear of being "found out."

Feels separate, double, divided into two parts.

Fears going mad, losing control, and leaving the body.

Feels that someone is trying to possess him or her, making the person "do" things.

Stiffness and cracking of joints; worse in cold, damp weather. Feels the legs are made of wood.

Gets stuck in depression; feels nothing will change; tired of life; upset by slightest contradiction or difficulty; sensitive and impressionable; music makes the person cry.

Feels as though he or she has committed a crime; worries about the future; fearful of salvation.

Sleep disturbed by amorous or frightful dreams, or dreams of falling from a height.

Wakes at 3.00 am and unable to get back to sleep.

Excessive production of tissue, mucus, or sweat.

Cysts or styes on the eyelids; warty growths; skin tags; polyps; fibroids; cysts of all sorts.

Inflammations and discharges from the genital area, usually yellowish-green and offensive; sweaty.

Left-sided complaints. Desires cold drinks, salt, and tea.

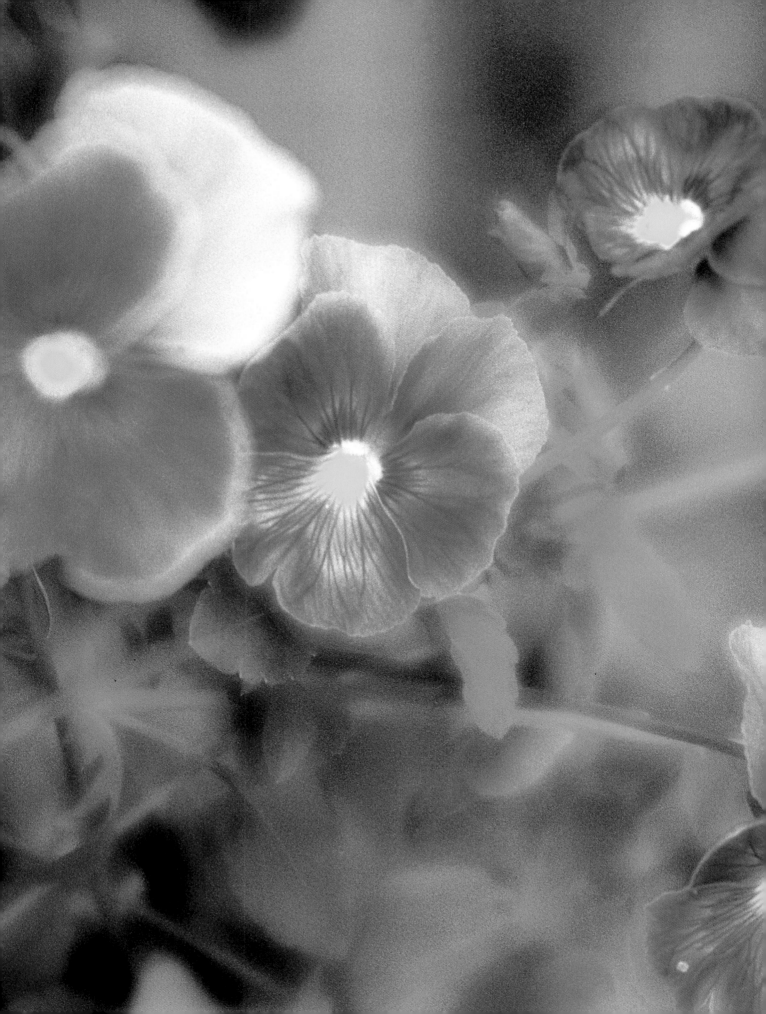

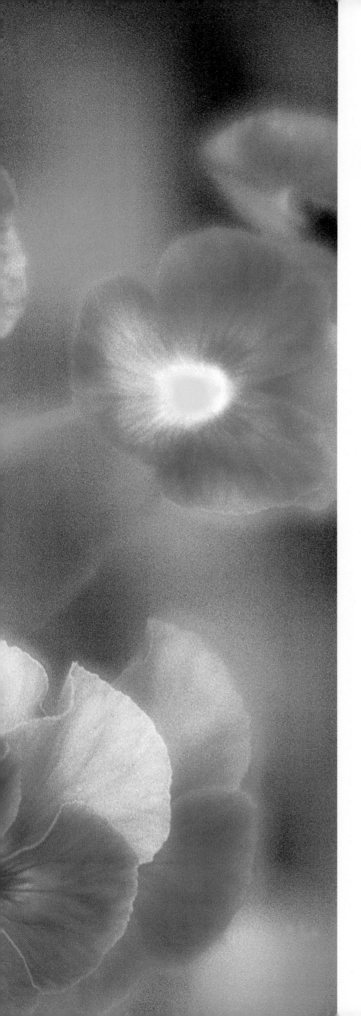

Directory
of common
ailments

In this section, some of the most common family illnesses and conditions are listed alphabetically, along with a selection of the best remedies to treat the condition. When you have looked under what you wish to treat and found an appropriate remedy, go back to the *Materia Medica* for more details about your choice.

Directory of common ailments

In this section we have selected certain common and well-known conditions for treatment. We have used the names of the conditions or illnesses, listed some of the best remedies, and specified the most characteristic, distinguishing symptoms.

To use this directory, look at the named condition and the remedies suggested for it, then look up the pictures of those remedies in the *Materia Medica* (see pages 38–71). Check to see if the characteristics described in the remedy picture match the characteristics of the sick person well enough to prescribe that particular remedy.

If the remedy suggested does not help the person, go back to the *Materia Medica* and see whether one of the other profiles fits better, whether or not that profile includes the named condition. You can use a remedy where the picture suits the person, even if the person's condition is not named in this section, because homeopathy treats the person, not the illness.

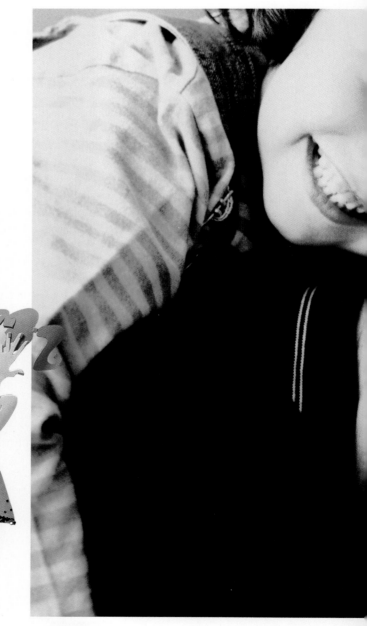

ABSCESSES, BOILS, WHITLOWS

Belladonna: for red, hot, shining skin; throbbing, burning pain; use before pus forms.

Hepar sulf: for early stages of pus formation; severe pain, sensitivity to cold and touch.

Silica: for chronic, septic states that are slow to develop, or at the end of the process.

Belladonna is useful for treating boils before pus forms and where there is red, hot, shining skin.

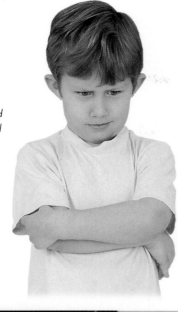

Chamomilla is very good for easing irritability and anger in children.

Staphysagria is an effective remedy for resentment and suppressed anger in people who are normally restrained and compliant.

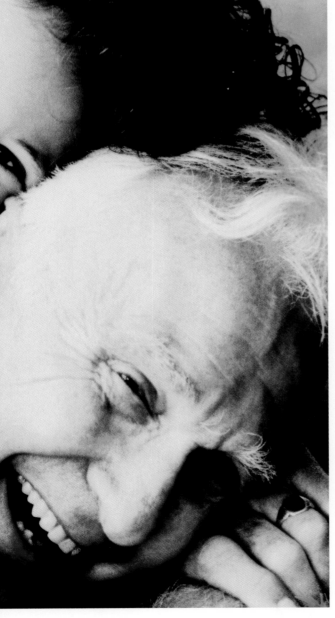

ANGER, IRRITABILITY

Arsenicum: for cold, self-righteous anger; critical and censorious attitude, and righteous indignation; impulses to stab and kill.

Chamomilla: for a child's anger; intolerable rage..

Ignatia: for short-lived spasms of anger from stress; for quarrelsome or "hysterical" behavior.

Lachesis: for passionate, uninhibited anger; revengeful feelings; talkativeness; feeling worse before periods and during menopause.

Lycopodium: for tyrannical behavior and verbal bullying; irritability and impatience; sudden explosions of temper; tendency to pick quarrels.

Nux vomica: for spasms of anger, and quick, uncontrollable temper; irritability; intolerance of contradiction; tendency to throw things.

Sepia: for bad temper; desire to leave home; spite; intolerance of contradiction; overwork.

Staphysagria: for suppressed anger and resentment, with occasional outbursts, in normally restrained, compliant person.

ALLERGIC REACTION

Apis: for sudden swelling of tongue or tissues of throat, from whatever cause.

Arsenicum: for breathing difficulties and suffocation (often from animal hair).

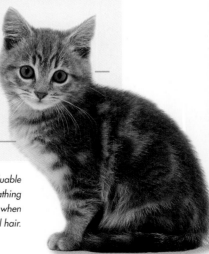

Arsenicum is a valuable remedy for breathing difficulties, especially when caused by animal hair.

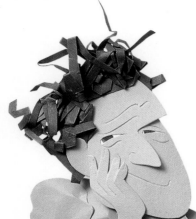

For a person who is anxious, restless, and cannot be reassured, the remedy Arsenicum could be helpful.

ASTHMA

Arsenicum: for anxiety and restlessness, wheezing, and burning sensations in chest; when worse for lying down; prostration; worse for pollen, animal hair, and at midnight –3.00 am.

Ipecac: for sudden onset of wheezing, feeling of suffocation, and weight on chest; constant rattling cough but cannot bring up any mucus; nausea.

Nux vomica: for attack after stomach upset; irritability.

Phosphorus: for noisy, wheezy breathing in tall, thin, anxious person.

Note: chronic asthma should always be treated by a homeopath.

ANXIETY

(including panic, claustrophobia, agoraphobia, other phobias and fears)

Aconite: for sudden onset of symptoms, and from shock and fear.

Argentum nitricum: for extremely anxious sense of anticipation, with nervous diarrhea and flatulence; worse for heat; hurried, flustered, and agitated behavior.

Arsenicum: for extreme anxiety, restlessness, and when person cannot be reassured; for paralyzing sense of weakness and obsessional behavior.

Gelsemium: for anxious anticipation; anxiety about performance; low spirits; weak and tremulous; paralysed with anxiety; nervous diarrhea.

Lycopodium: for hypochondriacal anxiety; fear of all illness, especially cancer; when anxious about performance, but performs well.

Pulsatilla: for timid, emotional, indecisive behavior; craving reassurance, or crying or fainting easily.

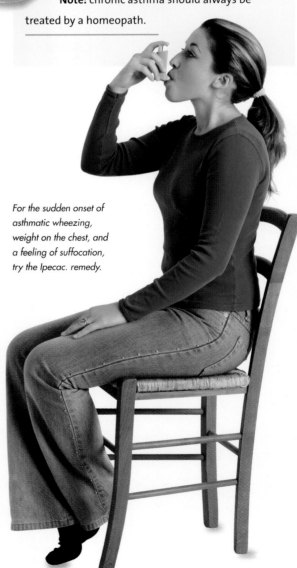

For the sudden onset of asthmatic wheezing, weight on the chest, and a feeling of suffocation, try the Ipecac. remedy.

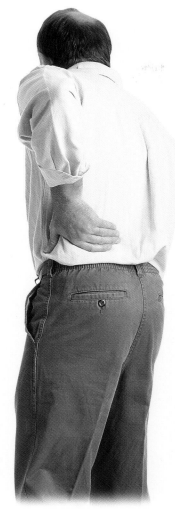

Use Arnica for backache caused by a long period of sitting or traveling. It is also useful for backache caused by injury.

BLEEDING

Arnica: for injury with shock; shock.

Belladonna: for nosebleeds caused by congestion; throbbing headache; red face.

China: with weakness; dim vision, ringing ears.

Ipecac: for gushes of bright-red blood, as in nosebleeds, with severe nausea and cold sweat.

Lachesis: for headache; flushing, cold extremities; fatigue; menstrual flooding; feelings of suspicion.

Phosphorus: for profuse nosebleed; heavy periods.

Sepia: for menstrual flooding with bearing-down pain; backache; for a feeling of womb falling out.

BACKACHE

Arnica: for after injury, long period of sitting or traveling, or bruised pain.

Rhus tox: for exposure to cold; when feeling better for heat and motion, yet worse for first movement.

Sepia: for dragged-down feeling; when worse for sitting and better for pressure; constipation, irritability; during pregnancy; menopause.

BED WETTING

Arsenicum: for an overconscientious, anxious, and chilly child.

Gelsemium: for a nervous, excitable child, with a sense of anxious anticipation or excitement.

BURNS

Keep *Cantharis* ointment and tablets handy in the kitchen. Best remedy for burns.

Arnica: for serious burns with shock; collapse.

Apis: for burning, stinging swelling, as if pricked by hot needles; relieved by cold compresses.

Belladonna: with swellings, especially when red, shiny, inflamed, and hot, with throbbing pain.

COLIC

Chamomilla: with twisting pain; diarrhea, especially at night; irritability; when symptoms are better for localized heat.

Nux vomica: with severe cramps; flatulence; spasmodic pains; when better for sitting or lying down.

CONSTIPATION AND DIARRHEA

Arsenicum: with anxiety, chilliness, and weakness; nausea and vomiting; watery, green or pale diarrhea from eating spoiled food or excessive fruit; food poisoning.

Bryonia: with irritability and bad temper; large, hard, dry stools, dark as if burned, and passed with great difficulty; *Bryonia* is often useful for children.

China: with weakness; pale, slimy diarrhea, with mucus; painless, but with weakness and severe flatulence; too much milk, fruit, and gluten.

Gelsemium: with nervousness and excitement; diarrhea from anticipation; fear; trembling.

Nux vomica: with impatience; ineffectual urging to pass stools; itching piles; and diarrhea caused by overeating.

Pulsatilla: with weepiness; stools variable, but worse in the evening; after starchy or fatty food.

Sulfur: with ineffectual urging to pass stools; hard, dry, dark stools; at other times, stools are yellow and watery, or slimy and with undigested food; urgent need drives person from bed at 5.00 am; anal fissure.

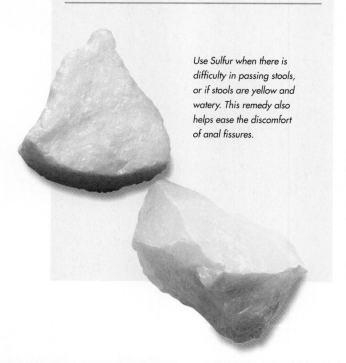

Use Sulfur when there is difficulty in passing stools, or if stools are yellow and watery. This remedy also helps ease the discomfort of anal fissures.

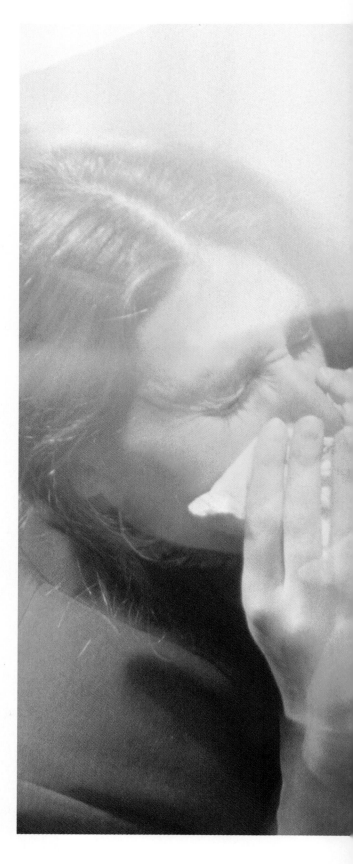

COUGHS, COLDS AND INFLUENZA

Aconite: for early stages after exposure to cold; anxiety and restlessness; feverish, flushed face; feeling worse at night; frequent sneezing; burning throat; thirst; dry, hard cough and croup; worse entering a warm room.

Arsenicum: restlessness, irritability, and anxiety; thin, watery nasal discharge, skin from the nostrils and the upper lip; burning pains, better for heat; hot drinks; dry cough; head colds that go to chest; thirst for sips of water; influenza.

Belladonna: for sudden onset of symptoms; feverish, flushed red face; skin feels hot and dry to the touch; sore throat is bright red, worse right side, and burns; pain on swallowing; dry, tickling, teasing cough, cough worse at night; infrequent thirst; sensitivity to light; throbbing headache.

Bryonia: with irritability, desire to be left alone; when cold goes to chest quickly; cough hard and dry with pains in throat and chest; feels better for sitting up, but worse when going from cold to warm; worse for the slightest movement: dry lips and mouth; very thirsty for cold drinks; persistent chest problems, bronchitis, and influenza.

Causticum: for hoarseness and dryness in the throat and chest, which are usually worse in the morning; hollow, irritating cough; laryngitis.

Gelsemium: with need to be left alone; sluggishness, apathy, and indifference to life; gradual onset of symptoms; heavy feeling in eyes and limbs; aches and pains; chilly feeling; dull headache; feverish, red face; seldom thirsty; major remedy for influenza.

Ipecac: for dry, teasing, spasmodic, and suffocating cough, with nausea and vomiting, or nosebleeds; mucus in bronchial tubes and lungs; bronchitis; worse for damp or sudden changes in weather.

Kali carb.: for a tendency to catch colds; when hard, white mucus flies out of mouth while coughing; severely catarrhal states, which turn to bronchitis or pneumonia if left unchecked.

Merc sol.: cold begins with creeping chilliness, much sneezing, and raw, smarting nostrils; thick, yellow-green nasal discharge or profuse irritating watery discharge; painful swallowing; throat hot and dry.

Nux vomica: for person who is irritable and easily offended; sudden onset of chilliness, sneezing spells; nose runny during daytime, yet congested at night; sore throat; dry, teasing cough, which is often painful in spells; worse for cold and open air; better for lying down and warmth.

Phosphorus: for colds that go to chest; weakness; thirst for ice-cold drinks, but may vomit as soon as water warms in stomach; laryngitis with or without pain (may lose voice); hoarseness, which is worse in the evening.

Pulsatilla: for stuffy nose at night and indoors, and which flows in open air; thick, creamy yellow discharge; cough dry in the evening, and loose in the morning; lips chapped and peeling; thirstless, despite fever; chilly, craves open air and is better for it; weepy and wants attention.

CROUP

Aconite: in first stage of symptoms, when the cough is dry, loud, and barking, and the child is restless and anxious.

Spongia: in second stage, if symptoms persist and child's breathing is harsh and hard.

Hepar sulf: in third stage, when the cough is loose and rattling, and has a deeper tone.

CYSTITIS

Arsenicum: with burning pains, which are better for hot applications.

Cantharis: with severe stinging pains, before, during, and after urination; when urination is frequent, but only small quantities are passed, which are often bloody.

Staphysagria: for after sexual activity.

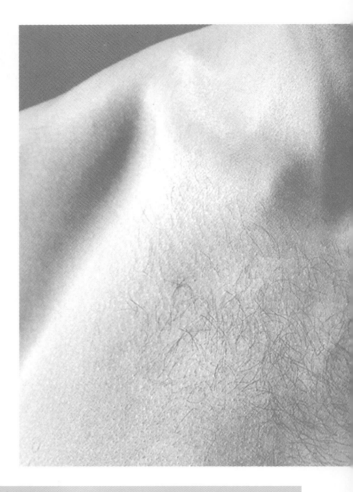

DEPRESSION

Arsenicum: with agitation, where the person's more anxious than depressed; for anxiety about health and when the person despairs of recovery; self-reproach, convinced of having offended friends; blames others; guilt; symptoms worse at midnight.

Aurum met.: with passivity; melancholy; blaming circumstance and fate rather than others; feels better for classical music; for symptoms caused by loss— business loss and disappointment in love; suicidal: worries and plans and then does it on impulse.

Ignatia: after loss, grief, or the break-up of a relationship; quiet, withdrawn, and visibly struggling to control feelings or obviously distressed.

Lachesis: the person betrayed, trusts no-one, and fears people are out to get him or her; complete hopelessness, apathy, and longing for death; grief, loss caused by failure of enterprise; menopause; exaggerated mood swings; heavy drinking.

Natrum mur.: for deep, long-lasting depressive state, and feeling of resignation; person bottles-up feelings and rejects false sympathy; person prefers to be alone.

Sepia: for the person who shows no interest in anything: work, family, friends, or sex; the person cannot be bothered and feels dragged down; useful when this state arises after giving birth, overwork, exhaustion, viral infection, and during menopause.

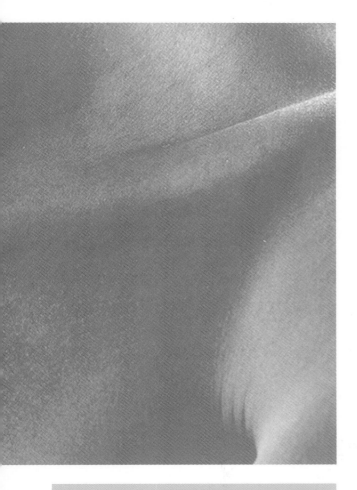

EARACHE

Aconite: with anxiety and fear; sudden onset after exposure to cold; ear red, hot, and painful, but better for warmth on affected area.

Belladonna: with sudden onset of symptoms, especially in the right ear; dry, flushed face and burning skin; symptoms better for heat, and worse for jarring movement; lack of thirst; frequent headaches.

Chamomilla: with irritability and anger; feels better when carried; one cheek red and hot, the other pale and cold; pain unbearable and is worse for heat on affected part.

Merc. sol.: for earache in damp, changeable weather, worse at night; person is sweaty and smells sick; profuse saliva and bad breath; worse in a warm bed; sensation of ice-cold water in ear.

Pulsatilla: for a person who is weepy and wants sympathy; throbbing pains come and go, and ears feel stopped up; catarrh; fever; worse for warmth and wants fresh air; feels worse in the evening and at night; glue ear.

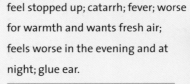

Pulsatilla is a very good remedy for earache in a child, when the throbbing pains come and go and the child is weepy and needs sympathy.

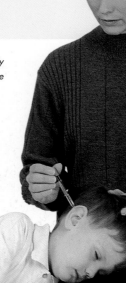

ECZEMA

Sulfur: for rough, irritable skin; often infected, is worse for water and the heat of bed; cracks in skin.

Rhus tox.: for blisters and skin irritation; better for heat; worse at night.

Note: it is always best to consult a homeopath about eczema and other skin diseases.

FALL AND INJURIES

Arnica: for bruising or pain resulting from a fall; sprain or any injury; take as soon as possible.

Hypericum: for when nerves are affected.

Ignatia is helpful for a person with a range of symptoms associated with grief, including sighs, tears, anxiety, fear, and silent, inexpressible sadness.

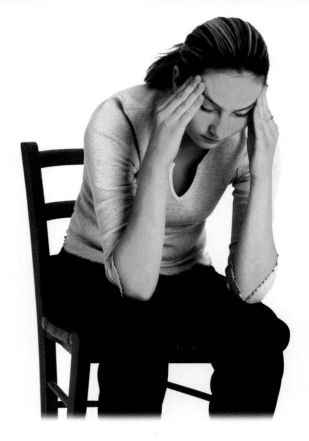

GRIEF AND LOSS

Aconite: for when death comes as a shock; when panic is the strongest feeling.

Causticum: for a person who grieves for others as much as for self; where anxiety and confusion follow bereavement.

Ignatia: with many symptoms of grieving: sighs, tears, laughter, anger, anxiety, fear, "hysteria," or silent, inexpressible sadness.

Natrum mur.: for grief endured for a long time; strong sense of having had something precious stolen from them; for when sympathy aggravates.

Pulsatilla: for silent grief; need for constant support, reassurance, and consolation.

Staphysagria: for reserved grief; difficulty expressing anger with loss.

HAY FEVER

Arsenicum: with restlessness and anxiety; thin, burning, excoriating, watery discharge, which is worse midnight–3.00 am.

Kali carb.: with symptoms that are worse indoors, and better for open air; symptoms worse in the morning and evening; upper eyelids swollen; thick discharge, which is clear or yellow.

Also *Mixed pollen* or *Allium cepa* might be helpful, or a potentized preparation of the substance causing the hay fever.

HEADACHE

Belladonna: for burning, throbbing, congestive headache, with sudden onset; worse for light, noise, and jarring movement; flushed face; head better for warmth.

Ignatia: for when there is a sensation of a band around the forehead; for a person who is emotional or who is holding in strong emotion; "hysterical" behavior; after upset, grief, or loss.

Nux vomica: for headache after eating, when accompanied by constipation; headache worse in the morning, after overindulgence in food or drink; hangover; irritability and hyperactivity.

Pulsatilla: for a weepy person, who needs support; pain throbbing and variable; symptoms better for cold applications and open air.

Lachesis: in menopause; for woman who feels worse before periods; throbbing headache, worse after sleep, but better for discharge and once menstrual flow is established.

HEART EPISODE/HEART ATTACK

Call the doctor immediately, and while waiting, try one of the following remedies.

Aconite: for severe attack, at the first onset of the symptoms.

Arsenicum: for a thin, tense, obsessional person, who is chilly and overanxious.

Nux vomica: for impatient, ambitious, self-driving person; irritability.

INSECT BITES AND STINGS

Apis: for any sting with local swelling and redness.

Arnica: for where there is shock, but less swelling and redness than *Apis*.

Staphysagria: for midge or mosquito bites. Try taking a low dose over a period of ten days before the start of the season. This seems to raise the immunity and give protection from attack.

INSOMNIA

Aconite: after shock or panic, with restlessness and nightmares; fear of dying.

Arnica: for when person is too tired to sleep; fidgety; bed feels hard; jet lag.

Arsenicum: for restlessness, worry, apprehensiveness, foreboding dreams, wakes at midnight–2. oo am.

Chamomilla: for children who are wide awake and irritable, who want to be carried, or who are in pain.

Lycopodium: when mind is active; going over things of the day, waking around 4.00 am; dreaming, talking, and laughing in sleep.

Nux vomica: insomnia from studying; overindulgence in food or alcohol; waking at 3.00 am, then falling asleep just as it is time to get up.

For insomnia that is caused by apprehension, worry, restlessness, and a sense of foreboding, try Arsenicum.

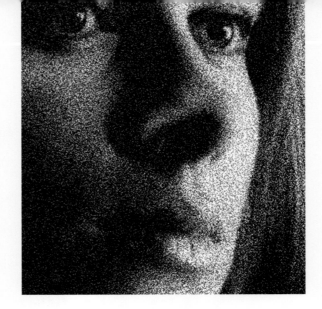

MENOPAUSE

Difficulties associated with the menopause are neither illnesses nor minor. You should consult a homeopath for help with this time of adjustment. All symptoms can be eased with various remedies. These two remedy pictures will show the potential.

Lachesis: hot flushes, fainting, flooding, melancholy, and weakness are all marked; profuse sweats, violent left-sided headaches, left-sided ovarian pain may be present; is worse after sleep, and worse when flow is delayed or suppressed; tendency to suspiciousness, jealousy, and rage may become distressing; no lessening of sexual interest.

Sepia: this remedy is associated with lack of muscular tone and congestion of blood in the veins; menopause accompanied by hot flushes, fainting, and anxiety; may be bleeding between periods; intense bearing-down sensation (as if everything would fall out) with pain in lower back; possible prolapse of womb and vagina; dryness and itching of vagina; pain on intercourse; loss of interest in sex.

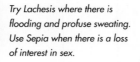

Try Lachesis where there is flooding and profuse sweating. Use Sepia when there is a loss of interest in sex.

MOUTH ULCERS

Merc. sol.: for foul breath and saliva; tongue that retains imprint of teeth; burning ulcers.

Natrum mur: for irritability; woman wants to be by herself; marked fluid retention; migraines.

Nux vomica: for irritability and anger, where woman is trying to get everything done, yet has no energy; constipation, and craving for candies or fatty foods.

Pulsatilla: for an irritable, touchy, weepy woman who needs reassurance; nausea with fainting, headaches, and back pain.

Sepia: for an irritable, angry woman, who wants to run away from home; depression; total lack of interest in sex; craving for sweets or salty foods.

SHOCK

Aconite: with agitation, restlessness, and fearfulness; if shock is primarily emotional.

Arnica: for shock that is mainly physical, due to injury or accident.

NAUSEA AND VOMITING

Arsenicum: for upset caused by eating spoiled food, especially bad meat; burning pains in stomach relieved by warm drinks; person chilly and anxious.

Ipecac: for persistent violent nausea, which is not relieved by vomiting; profuse saliva; feeling of disgust for all types of food.

Nux vomica: with irritability; wakefulness after 3.00 am; upset caused by spicy, rich food, or too much food and drink; desire to vomit, but inability to do so.

Phosphorus: with great thirst for cold water, which is vomited when it becomes warm in stomach.

Pulsatilla: person who is chilly and weeping; symptoms worse for starchy, fatty food, especially butter and cream; dry mouth, but not thirsty.

Nux vomica: for irritability and anger, where woman is still trying to get everything done, yet has no energy; constipation, and craving for sweet or fatty foods.

Pulsatilla: for an irritable, touchy, weepy woman who needs reassurance; nausea, headaches and back pain.

PREMENSTRUAL TENSION AND PAINFUL PERIODS

Calc. carb: for a timid, nervous, and self-conscious woman; craving for eggs and sweet things.

Lachesis: for a woman who is suspicious and angry; worse after sleep, and worse for tight clothing; dramatically better after bleeding starts.

Natrum mur: for irritability; woman wants to be by herself; marked fluid retention; migraines.

Nux vomica: for irritability and anger, where woman is still trying to get everything done, yet has no energy; constipation, and craving for sweet or fatty foods.

Pulsatilla: for an irritable, touchy, weepy woman who needs reassurance; nausea with fainting, headaches, and back pain.

Sepia: for an irritable, angry woman, who wants to run away from home; depression; total lack of interest in sex; craving for candies or salty foods.

Bryonia: for symptoms that are worse for heat.

RHEUMATISM AND ARTHRITIS

Bryonia: for symptoms that are worse for heat and movement, especially jarring movement; better for rest and cool applications.

Causticum: for symptoms that are better for warmth, and are unaffected by movement; better for rain; jaw and neck affected, and stiff neck.

Rhus tox: for burning tearing pains; better for heat and continued movement; worse for sitting, rest, first movement, cold, and damp.

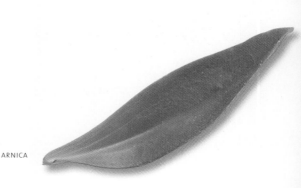

ARNICA

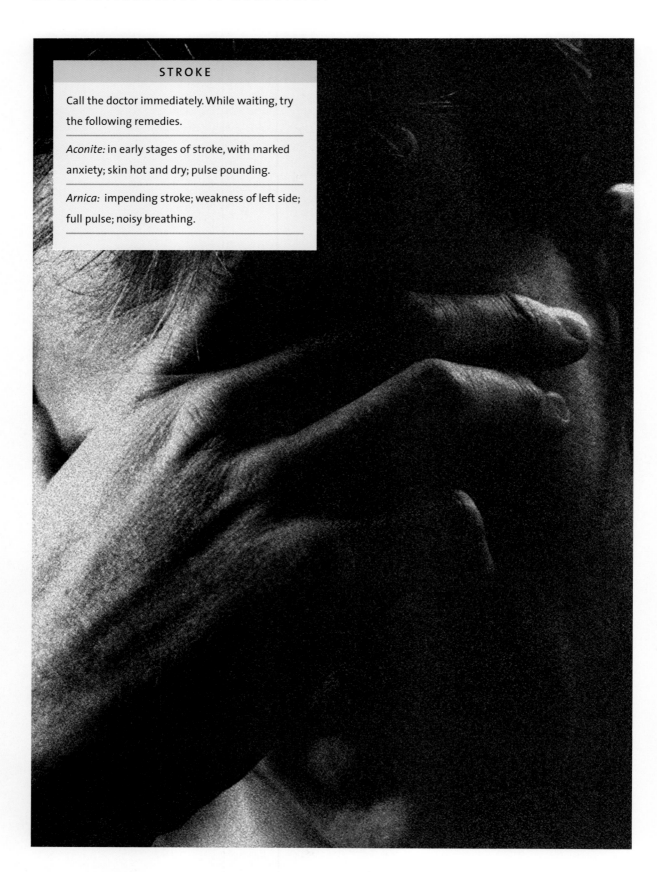

STROKE

Call the doctor immediately. While waiting, try the following remedies.

Aconite: in early stages of stroke, with marked anxiety; skin hot and dry; pulse pounding.

Arnica: impending stroke; weakness of left side; full pulse; noisy breathing.

SUNSTROKE OR EFFECTS OF THE SUN

Belladonna: with pupils that are dilated and bloodshot; strong pulse; where there is a pounding, bright-red face; skin burning, dry, and flushed; high body temperature.

TONSILLITIS

Belladonna: right-sided; redness and swelling; neck stiff; throat red and dry; painful to swallow; worse for drinking liquids; hot, congested head; profuse sweats.

Merc. sol.: for painful, dry throat, with frequent pus discharge; white spots or false membrane covering throat; tongue swollen; profuse saliva; intense thirst; foul breath.

TOOTHACHE

Aconite: from cold wind; better for cold water.

Belladonna: with stabbing, throbbing pain in gums; inflammation, with headache.

Chamomilla: in teething problems and pains.

Merc. sol.: with stabbing pains radiating to ears; a lot of salivation; worse at night.

Staphysagria: with teeth sensitive to the least touch and cold air; tearing pains, which are worse at night.

VACCINATION

Thuja: for bad effects of vaccination.

VARICOSE VEINS, INFLAMED

Aconite: with inflammation caused by long periods of walking, traveling, or flying.

Arnica: with tenderness, which is worse when touched.

Belladonna: for when the area has become hot, red, and tender and is throbbing.

Lachesis: for blueish/violet veins; hypersensitivity to touch; throbbing pain, which is better for bleeding, and worse for heat.

Sepia: for sagging; congestion of veins.

WOUNDS

Apply *Hypercal* or *Calendula* tincture externally.

Hepar sulf.: for the early stages of infection, where there is pus and intense pain on touch. Foreign bodies, such as splinters and rose thorns, will be ejected.

Silica: for when the infection and pus linger.

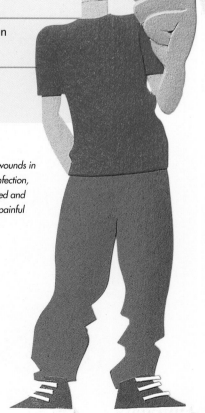

Use Hepar sulf. for wounds in the early stages of infection, where pus has formed and the affected area is painful to the touch.

Case histories

These case histories are examples of how homeopathy can help a range of ailments. From sore throats and bronchitis to food poisoning, the examples here demonstrate the value of homeopathic treatment in the home or by a professional.

CASE HISTORY 1

A young student came to see me. He was getting irritated and angry easily, especially after a night out. He had hit a wall the previous Saturday, because, he said, he would have hit his girlfriend otherwise. He was going to bed late, waking early in the morning, lying sleepless, then falling asleep just when it was time to get up. He was picking quarrels with his friends, and flying off the handle about the slightest thing. He was constipated and always wanting chocolate. He admitted he was worrying about the amount of alcohol he was drinking. He had to sit final exams in a few months and was doing a lot of work.
Nux vomica was clearly indicated. After treatment with it, he was able to control his drinking and temper much more easily. The constipation and sleeplessness also improved.

CASE HISTORY 2

A patient who was due to take her driving test was terrified and anticipating failure. She had constant diarrhea and felt paralyzed with anxiety. She was given *Gelsemium 30* to take as needed. When she returned, she reported that she had not only passed her driving test easily, but had caught herself singing round the house before going to the Test Center.

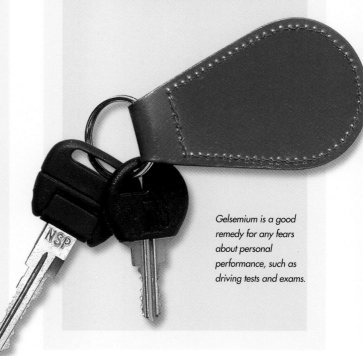

Gelsemium is a good remedy for any fears about personal performance, such as driving tests and exams.

CASE HISTORY 3

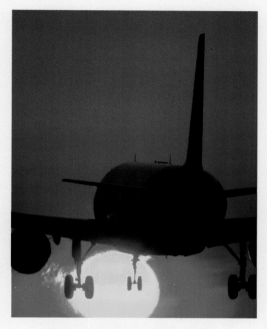

Use Argent. nit. for fears of flying, heights and tall buildings, enclosed spaces and crowds, being alone, and illness and death.

Another woman, who was afraid of traveling by air, had been given *Argent. nit. 30* to take as needed before a trip to Spain. Before flying, she normally became very agitated and on edge. After taking the remedy the day before and on the morning of the flight, she remained calm, even though the plane was delayed for several hours, due to unspecified "mechanical failure." In fact, she gave her spare remedies to other panicking travelers and probably averted a mass panic.

CASE HISTORY 4

A boy of nine was brought to a homeopath because he kept being off school with colds, sore throats, and swollen glands. He had chilly, sweaty hands and sweated profusely around his head at night. He had had a lot of high fevers when younger and had never slept well. He would often scream in his sleep and tell his mother of terrifying dreams. Recently he had revealed that he was being bullied at school and other boys called him names. After a high potency of *Calc. carb.*, the boy improved in his overall health. He had no more colds that winter and started to stand up for himself at school.

CASE HISTORY 5

There is a famous story of how one of the early homeopaths became convinced of the healing power of homeopathy when he gave *Sepia* to a ewe that refused to look after her newborn lambs. Immediately after having been given the *Sepia*, she ambled over to them and placidly let them suck.

CASE HISTORY 6

Once, I had a patient who was looking for help with recurring bronchitis. She had red hair and a wiry stature. In the course of the first interview, she told me that she had met a man from Pluto and talked to him. She had also solved the difficulties of homeopathic prescribing at home by giving her children all the homeopathic remedies in her kit at once, on the grounds that one of them would work. She had stopped wearing a watch because her body's electricity interfered with the workings of the watch. All these were superb indications for the suitability of *Phosphorus* and it improved her bronchitis enormously.

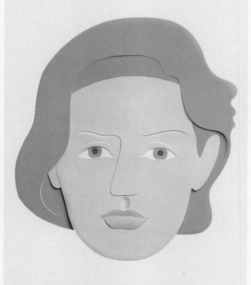

The Phosphorus remedy is excellent for easing bronchitis, mental fatigue, and irrational fears and imaginings.

CASE HISTORY 7

Marian was 15 years old, fair-haired, and blue-eyed. She had been extremely moody for several months. Her periods had not started until she was 14 years old: she had had one, then nothing for about three months; then a period, then nothing for a couple of months, then a few in a row and then nothing for three months. When she did have them, they were painful. She was worried. She cried quite a lot while telling me this. She hated fatty foods and they made her get indigestion. She was inclined to get catarrhal colds. What else could I give her but a high potency of *Pulsatilla*? Her periods settled into a steady pattern from then on and she became much more settled, contented, and happy.

Pulsatilla proved to be the right remedy to help treat painful, erratic periods and catarrhal colds.

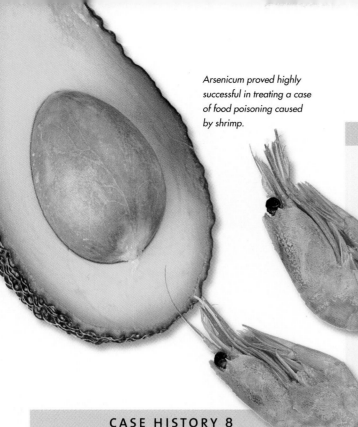

Arsenicum proved highly successful in treating a case of food poisoning caused by shrimp.

CASE HISTORY 9

A 35-year-old woman came to me with premenstrual tension, painful periods, and nausea. She had suffered from this since her teenage years. She reported that she got into a desperate state when she was hungry, but didn't eat much. She had swollen upper eyelids; they had always been like that. She suffered from backache sometimes, and the ligaments were weak. After being prescribed *Kali carb. 30c*, she had no more trouble for years.

CASE HISTORY 8

Mrs Allen rang in the morning. She had been vomiting and having diarrhea since about 3.00 am. She looked green and felt sick. She had been out to dinner the night before and had chosen avocado with shrimp. She had had her suspicions at the time: she should have been more careful, she said, but her husband had said it was alright. She was shivering and very anxious, thinking she had eaten something fatal. Could it be *E. coli*? *Arsenicum 6c* every half and hour was prescribed until improvement was felt, then gradually less often. She rang in the afternoon to say that she had felt less anxious almost immediately and recovered from the sickness in the course of the day.

CASE HISTORY 10

June was normally a very active, hardworking woman of about forty. Then she started to experience premenstrual tension and suffered from painful periods with backache. She was extremely depressed at these times, and felt as if someone had "pulled the plug out," She just wanted to slob around and stay in bed. The family avoided her because she would scream at them for no apparent reason. *Sepia* was prescribed successfully and June recovered.

CASE HISTORY 11

A woman came with a dry, stuffy cold and a harsh cough. She had had it for three or four weeks and it had not completely gone away. She was also suffering from pain in the knees. She was irritable with it and did not want to go for walks. Repeated doses of *Bryonia* in low potencies cleared up the troublesome cold and relieved the pain in the knees.

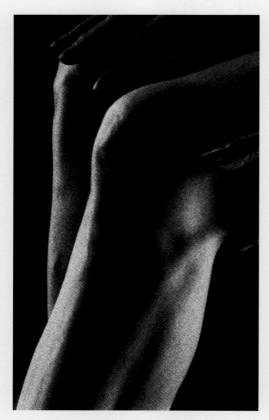

Bryonia provides welcome relief from the pain of injuries to knees and other joints, and when they are worse from moving.

CASE HISTORY 12

A patient had suffered a terrible earache for over 24 hours. It had come on suddenly after she had been burgled. She had tried *Belladonna*, which had always worked for her earache before, but *Belladonna* and painkillers had not done anything this time. She was panicky and anxious. I gave her *Aconite* because of the panic, even though she insisted it was logical to feel panicky and anxious after being burgled. The earache cleared within minutes and did not return.

CASE HISTORY 13

A friend called with her seven-year-old child. The girl was in a terrible state. She was difficult, upset, and having tantrums. She was having trouble sleeping at night. They had just come back from abroad. One dose of *Chamomilla 30c* sorted out the problem.

Use the soothing qualities of Chamomilla to help soothe stressed children, especially those who cannot sleep or who are teething.

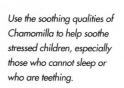

CASE HISTORY 14

My ginger tomcat, who was always very amiable and mild mannered, suddenly started to be very irritable and cross. I tried to find out what the matter was, but he just hissed and scratched. This was so unlike him that I gave him *Hepar sulph 30c* on account of his touchiness and temper. Within minutes of my giving it to him, pus poured from a septic wound on his face, which I had not seen because of his thick fur.

CASE HISTORY 15

A friend rang in the late afternoon, hardly able to speak. Her husband took the phone. She had just been stung in the mouth by a wasp, which had got into a can of lemonade she had been drinking. Her mouth and throat were swelling, and she could not move her tongue. They were both terrified. After *Apis 30c*, she went out to dinner as planned, with no discomfort.

CASE HISTORY 16

A young woman came to me complaining of extreme tiredness and weakness. She felt chilly and exhausted much of the time. She had been like this for a few months; in fact, she had never felt right since an abdominal operation. She had pain at the site of the wound sometimes. She was cautious and timid, but determined. I gave her *Silica* on the strength of the tiredness and her character. When she returned a month later, she was feeling much better and had been astonished to notice that, just a few days after being given the remedy, some black silk stitches came out of the wound.

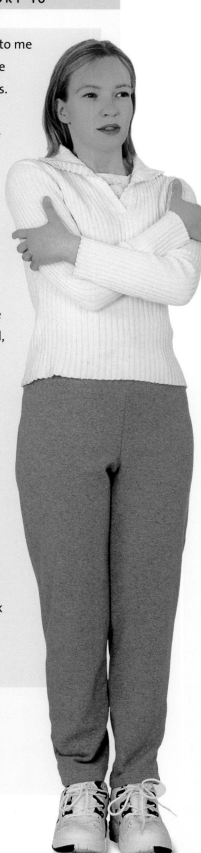

Silica promotes the expulsion of any foreign matter from the body, such as splinters and even stitches from wounds.

Useful addresses

American Institute of Homeopathy
801 North Fairfax Street
Suite 306
Alexandria
VA 22314

Council for Homeopathic Certification
1199 Sanchez Street
San Francisco
CA 94114

Hahnemann Homeopathic Pharmacy
828 San Pablo Avenue
Albany
California
CA 94706

Hahnemann Medical Clinic
1918 Bonita Ave.
Berkeley
CA 94704

Homeopathic Academy of Naturopathic Physicians
P.O. Box 12488
Portland
OR 97212

North American Society of Homeopaths (NASH)
1122 East Pike Street, # 1122
Seattle
WA 98122
nashinfo@aol.com

The National Center for Homeopathy
801 North Fairfax Street
Suite 306
Alexandria
VA 22314
nchinfo@igc.apc.org

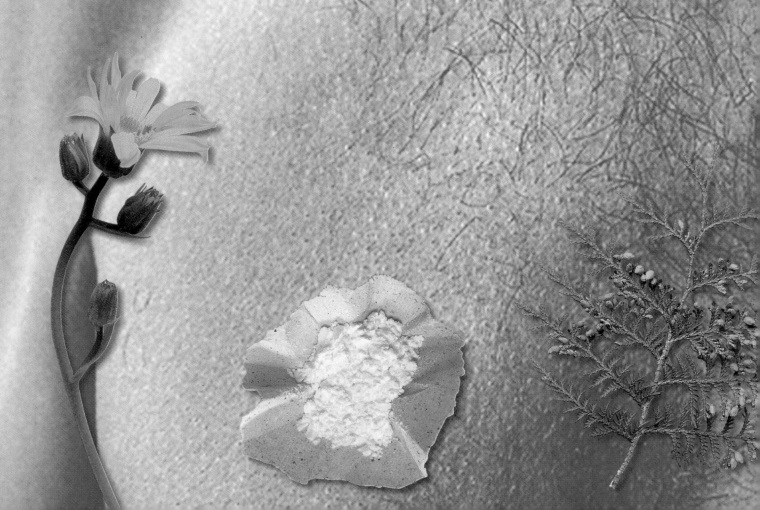

Index

abscesses 74
Aconite 26, 27, 34, 42
acute conditions 22–3
allergic reactions 75
anger 75
anxiety 76
Apis 43, 93
Argent nito 44, 89
Arnica 34, 45
Arsenicum 19, 31, 46, 91
asthma 76
Aurum met. 47

backache 77
bed wetting 77
Belladonna 26, 27, 28, 34, 48, 92
bites 83
bleeding 77
boils 74
Bryonia 31, 49, 92
burns 77

Calc. carb. 31, 50, 89
case histories 88–93
Causticum 51
Chamomilla 26, 34, 52, 92
China 31, 53
chronic conditions 22–3
colds 79
colic 77
constipation 78
constitutional types 20–1
coughs 79
croup 80
cystitis 80

depression 12, 80
diarrhea 78
dilution 14–15

earache 81
eczema 81

falls 81

Gelsemium 54, 88
grief 82

Hahnemann, Samuel 7–14
hay fever 82
headache 82
heart attack 83
Hepar sulf. 26, 31, 55, 93
homeopaths 22–3

Ignatia 56
influenza 79
injuries 81
insomnia 83
Ipecacuanha 57
irritability 75

Kali carb. 31, 58, 91

Lachesis 31, 59
loss 82
Lycopodium 60

Materia Medica 39–71
menopause 84
Merc. sol. 26, 61
mouth ulcers 85

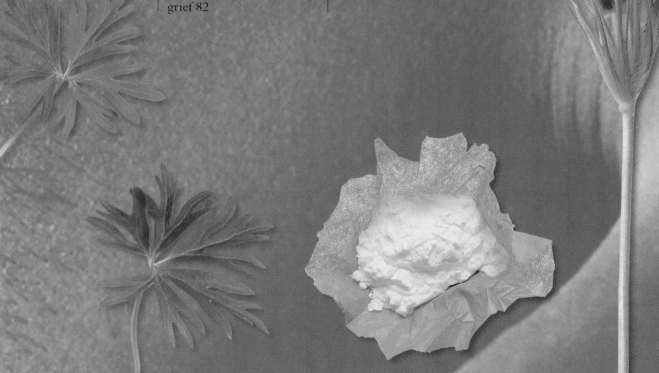

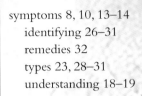

Natrum mur. 31, 62
nausea 85
Nux vomica 31, 63, 88

Phosphorus 31, 64, 90
potencies 14–15, 34, 36–7
Pulsatilla 19, 20–1, 26, 27, 28, 65, 90

remedies 8, 10, 12–15
   choosing 26–7
   complete picture 20–1
   finding 32
   giving 34–5

illness types 23
   taking 34–5
   understanding 18–19
   waiting 36–7
Rhus. tox. 66

Sepia 12, 67, 89, 91
shock 84
Silica 26, 68, 93
Staphysagria 69
stings 83
stroke 86
Sulfur 26, 31, 70
sunstroke 86

symptoms 8, 10, 13–14
   identifying 26–31
   remedies 32
   types 23, 28–31
   understanding 18–19

Thuja 71
tonsilitis 87
toothache 87

vaccination 87
varicose veins 87
vital force 11, 14
vomiting 85

whitlows 74
wounds 87

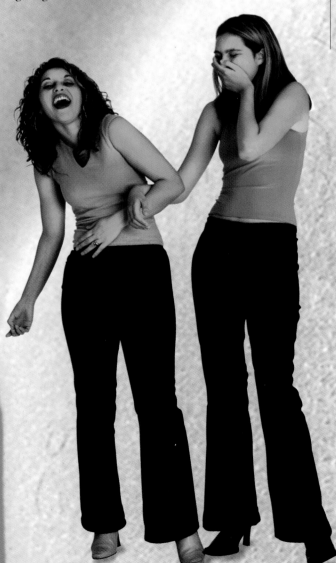

Acknowledgements

Special thanks go to
Jane Lanaway for design and
photography co-ordination
Malika Hopkins, Peter Donno,
Chloe Winter, Stephanie Winter,
and Ian Parsons for help
with photography

*The publishers would like to thank
the following for the use of pictures:*
A–Z Botanical Collection 49
Corbis 6/7 10/11 16/17 24/25
38/39 42 47 48 57 60 66
Image Bank 9 28 78/79
Images Colour Library 19 72/73
Stone Gettyone 1 20/21 52
74/75 89
Superstock 32/33
Trudi Valter for picture research